Senses and sensitivity

The 'doing' of Five Element
constitutional acupuncture

*How to fine-tune your sensory acuity
and emotion testing skills*

John Hicks

Laughing Water Press

'Listen with your ears.
No don't listen with your ears.
Listen with your mind.
No, don't listen with your
mind. Listen with your spirit.
The spirit is empty and waits
on all things.'

Zhuangzi, 369–266 BCE

Contents

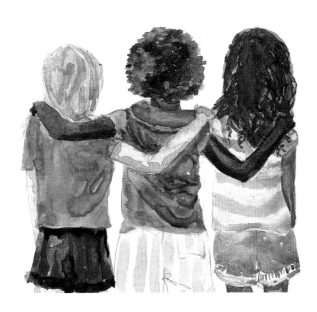

This book is respectfully dedicated to my first acupuncture teacher, JR Worsley. JR taught finding the 'causative factor' via colour, sound, emotion and odour. I studied in his college, completing his Lic Ac, BAc, MAc and – with three others – his Dr Ac course, and taught there for over ten years. My practice at that time was in the college clinic and JR was frequently available for consultations where I also observed him emotion testing. These moments were invaluable to me and gradually I began, with my NLP background, to model how he tested. Contact with him and receiving CF feedback from him changed my life.

Preface

In the history of Chinese medicine there have been multiple approaches to diagnosing and treating a person at the most basic level. Not just treating, for example, the after-effects of overeating or a brief infection, but treating at the constitution, so the patient at their basic core becomes stronger, more resilient and more balanced. Such treatment can't be fully separated from treating specific ailments and should also include advice on diet and lifestyle to support the constitutional treatment. Chinese medicine is a rich collection of approaches, but for me what gets called 'Five Element constitutional treatment', is special. Hence, this book.

It brings together under one cover the content of the Five Element Skills module I created for the College of Integrated Chinese Medicine (CICM) acupuncture degree course. Previously this material has only existed as handouts, and was taught verbally. The module is directed to the diagnostic skills required for practicing Five Element constitutional acupuncture. It is not so much about knowledge, but practical, sensory skills.

I hope *Senses and sensitivity* (with apologies to Jane Austen) will serve as a useful learning aid for students and for teachers of the CICM Skills module – and more widely students, teachers and practitioners anywhere who are curious about the details of what is loosely called the 'constitution' in Chinese medicine.

I have had two important supports whilst writing. One is my wife Angie with whom I have had endless 'book' discussions and the other is the teachers with whom I have co-taught various sessions, which has always reassured me the content and spirit of the material will be passed on.

1

Developing sensitivity in your practice

'We are what we repeatedly do. Excellence, then, is not an act, but a habit.'
Aristotle

'Skill is myelin insulation that wraps neural circuits and that grows according to certain signals.
The story of skill and talent is the story of myelin.'
Daniel Coyle, *The Talent Code*

Sensory acuity and emotional expressiveness

This book grew out of *Five Element Constitutional Acupuncture*.[1] In that textbook, Five Element constitutional acupuncture is explained in detail and Traditional Chinese Medicine (TCM) is explained briefly. Together these make a powerful curriculum.

The College of Integrated Chinese Medicine (CICM) combines the theory and the practice of Chinese medicine. That task requires a balance between **head learning** and developing both **sensory acuity** and **emotion testing skills**. My primary issue in this book is the initial and ongoing requirement to learn, stabilise and then develop the practitioner's sensory acuity (with colour, odour and sound) and the practitioner's ability to emotion test. That is, how to interact with the patient so as to reveal their 'least balanced' Five Element emotion.

Theory and practice require using both head and senses, but to varying degrees. Five Element theory is simple; its practice is more complex and requires the practitioner to develop their senses and an ability to be emotionally expressive. TCM relies more on head learning and questioning. This difference in emphasis is not absolute, but significant.

Five Element and TCM acupuncture have different strengths. Five Element practice focuses on strengthening the constitutional Element. This brings the Elements and emotions into greater balance and restores resilience and wellbeing. TCM focuses on the patient's main complaint and allows the practitioner to deal with the presenting symptoms. Five Element treatment requires a *sensory* focus in identifying the patient's colour, odour, sound and emotion and noticing pulse changes from treatment (and indeed sensitivity in the physical examination). Developing these sensitivities requires practice time, a small part of which is in class, but much of which is outside the classroom. TCM does not ignore sensory development but relies more on questioning signs and symptoms from Chinese medicine Organ functions, syndromes and differentiations of disease. Questioning efficiently is an important skill and also requires practise. As a generalisation, Five Element training requires more sensory learning and TCM requires more head learning. So?

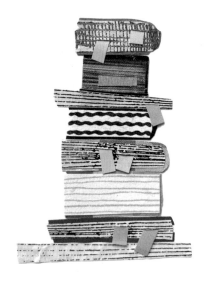

Head learning is typical of most academic courses. It *occurs* through lectures, reading books, making notes, writing assignments, talking to other students, or explaining to someone else the six functions of *qi* or the differences between Heart *yang* deficiency and Heart *yin* deficiency. Also, good teachers, good handouts and a good textbook help enormously. It is *assessed* through written exams.

Sensory learning is different. Five Element acupuncture requires close observation of the facial colour (somehow dealing with applied, artificial makeup colours), smelling people's Five Element odour (having separated out the many artificial perfume odours), and hearing the Five Element sounds in people's voices (compared with the content). It also includes how to interact with patients so that, Element by Element, the Five emotions are revealed – which requires expressive flexibility and simultaneous observation, which is different for each Element and requires a learning process as complex as learning to walk.

Sensory learning also includes pulse taking, both feeling the 15 basic pulse qualities and being able to monitor and evaluate pulse changes before and after each stage of treatment. Also important is a physical examination requiring a sensitive touch, a sensitive eye, a sensitive ear and a sensitive nose. The emphasis is less on knowledge, more on sensory acuity.

Course assessment is important as it influences a student's allocation of time. An academic course inclines towards the assessment of head learning. There are established test questions with model answers. The model answers are considered a sufficient test and very specific graded marks are given. In contrast, with acupuncture points and colour, odour, sound and emotion testing there is no similar, final practical test. Why? Point location assessment does not involve the needling of a point to discover whether *deqi* is obtained; nor does the assessment of the **constitutional factor (CF)** indicators involve a treatment test and feedback on the subsequent wellbeing or symptom improvement experienced by the patient. It is true that there is something approaching that when a student is in the clinic, but again the welfare of patients and the supervisors' assessment has priority. As a consequence, I believe that in the student's mind, academic success can easily trump practical success.

JR Worsley's approach to pulse taking was noticeably different from that practiced in China. In China, pulses are taken before treatment as part of the diagnosis, the qualities noted and not taken again. JR would take the pulses before treatment, record the volume/strength, note the degree of disharmony and then, after each phase of treatment, the pulses were taken again to *evaluate the change.* The criteria for change seemed to be:
- the different pulse positions became more similar, that is, in greater harmony
- the Element treated was less responsive than the others, suggesting that Element was the source of the imbalance in other Elements, and
- overall, the pulses felt more similar and (this word was not used) 'smoother'.

JR did not use the Chinese vocabulary of pulse qualities. Instead, he assessed them according to their change towards greater harmony.

In addition, JR rarely spoke about how he assessed a good pulse change, but I remember many instances on clinicals when he would glance at a patient who had been treated and, for him, that seemed enough.

He was assessing the change in the patient via a glance at the face. The student, and me as supervisor, were waiting for him to take the pulses and acknowledge the good change; but one glance at the face seemed to be all he needed. He was using the *look* of the patient: the sparkle in the eyes and a more alert, more balanced face. As JR's students gained experience, they tended to follow in his footsteps, rapidly reading small changes and judging improvement at a glance. But this teaching was implicit, not explicit.

At CICM we use JR's pulse approach, that is, more as feedback after each stage of treatment. But we also incorporate the main TCM pulse qualities for pre-treatment diagnosis – thereby achieving the best of both worlds. These pulse qualities are: depth, width, strength, shape, rhythm and rate, and their subcategories. These support the integrated diagnosis.

Until there is another JR – that is, someone willing and able to give absolutely correct feedback – practitioners and teachers must be willing to take risks, commit and let the results of treatment be the guide.

The evolving pattern of learning

Learning Five Elements on its own allowed more time and focus on sensory development. The integration of TCM has shifted the balance, unnoticed, to head learning from sensory acuity. Over time, the CICM teachers' backgrounds have changed. Those who taught at CICM in the early days practised just Five Elements, and only later learned TCM. TCM was a welcome addition to their practices. Now the majority of teachers are those who learned TCM and Five Elements together. There is less pressure on students to excel with colour, odour, sound and emotion testing, because it is hard to make sensory acuity objective and testable. This change has largely been unnoticed and partly explains the purpose of this book, how to work regularly on the:
- sensory awareness of colour, odour and sound
- emotion testing to find the emotion least in balance
- pulse taking to feel greater pulse harmony, and
- putting a priority on the mind and spirit as well as body.

Significantly, JR did not teach or explain emotion testing. He was a demonstrator, not an explainer. This book hopes to break down and thus explain the process.

Most graduate training does not, at this moment, fill the gap. It is often information-based and TCM oriented. Development of the senses can and should go on throughout one's career, but there is little guidance: for example, there is no external pressure after graduating to keep developing sensing. One of the purposes of this book is to encourage ongoing sensory development.

Why is sensory acuity and agreement such a big learning process?

We believe we live in a shared world, which we then assume is *the* world. We start to learn about this shared world as babies when we learn a language which then gets solidified as we develop into adults. We are encouraged to discover the *world we have in common,* more than our subjective worlds and we tend to end up believing that our shared world is *the* world. The development of language and print, designed so we can communicate, further solidifies our perception of the shared world and this world is again further solidified by the internet, books, radio, TV and our educational establishments.[2]

JR Worsley changed my view of this world even further, but in another way. I was told to diagnose patients using colour, odour, sound and emotion. That seemed sensible enough, but my perception of these was often different from JR's and then, when the results of his perception produced highly beneficial changes in the patients, I accepted what he said: that his students needed to re-learn to see, hear, smell and be aware of others' emotions.

Occasionally he was explicit, saying something like: 'I will teach you to see again'. I was in a kind of bind: I both took him seriously *and* I did not really know what he meant. But my sense of our shared world as *the* world fell into question.

Having been exclusively a Five Element acupuncturist for the first ten years of my practice, I and many colleagues' choice was simple: develop colour, odour, sound and emotion sensitivity or fail. Some, rather than fail, went on almost immediately to study TCM in order to survive. My choice, only after ten years of a busy Five Element practice, but based on some failures in the clinic, was to train in TCM in China. Why? There were a small number of patients with Full conditions (for instance pathogens such as Phlegm, Damp, Full Heat or Cold Blood or *qi* stagnation) who I failed to help. Up until that point I thought my senses were sufficient. What motivated me? My examples may well sound naïve today.

There was a lady in her 60s whose hands were swollen with Damp/ Phlegm. She said treatment made her feel better in herself, but did nothing for her hands. Her hands were the reason she'd sought treatment. She convinced me that a greater understanding of Fullness was essential. Also significant was a patient who was blocked with Phlegm and was misdiagnosed as having the Internal Dragons which failed to clear Phlegm. And I remember a Five Element graduate who had studied TCM early on, explaining to me how he had improved an ex-patient's health through clearing pathogens first and then treating the CF. I was grateful for that feedback.

Having learned TCM was helpful when treating Full conditions. I was better able to recognise Fullness and clear pathogens first, but with many patients Five Element treatment alone still seemed more effective.

I frequently found that these signs of Fullness were expelled by appropriate strengthening or Tonification and sometimes clearing pathogens. How to recognise if clearing a pathogen was essential was not obvious. So, protocols were developed to err on the side of caution.

For example: a patient is an Earth constitutional factor and has Damp. The Damp would be diagnosed, for example, because of lethargy, a slippery pulse, excess weight and swelling in the body. A choice arises: clear Damp first and only then Tonify Earth, possibly in sequence in the same treatment or in two or more treatments. With Wood CFs, the similar dilemma (involving, for example, Liver Blood deficiency and Liver qi stagnation, diagnosed mainly via a wiry pulse) could be resolved by using a smoothing technique (retaining the needles using even techniques) and assessing the pulse change while the needles were in. Learning to recognise pathogens, assessing if they need clearing and knowing how to do this became integrated and was an important learning.

Giovanni Maciocia discusses this issue from a TCM point of view in Chapter 69 of *The Foundations of Chinese Medicine*, pages 1171–89.[3] His answer (note his discussion on page 1186) is to treat Full and Empty conditions simultaneously, varying the needle technique according to treatment principle. I saw this practice carried out when in China. The solution described in Giovanni's book is: when in doubt, clear first and judge the importance of clearing via the pulse change. This procedure arose or was possible because of JR's use of pulse changes to evaluate treatment *as the treatment progressed.*

To be more specific, when in doubt about the degree of pathogen Fullness/*qi* stagnation and any need to use either even, reduction or a smoothing needle technique, the practitioner can smooth/clear first and use the accompanying pulse change to evaluate the need for clearing or strengthening. This procedure avoids any previous mistakes, for example, Tonifying when another needle technique was appropriate.

My current view is that in a majority of cases, Five Element treatment is basic and gets the best results in the shortest length of time. However, being able to recognise Full conditions via symptoms and pulses is essential, then smoothing/clearing/reducing, then re-assessing the priority of smoothing/clearing/reducing via the pulse change is beneficial, timesaving and safe. Encountering Full conditions, both acute and chronic, and knowing how to treat them is absolutely necessary.

So, for many of us, there was a new task: knowing how to recognise the presence of pathogens *and* whether they required clearing or would respond to CF strengthening. What I think requires emphasising is sufficient sensory training/practise to gain excellence with colour, odour, sound, emotion testing and reading pulses.

Three years' training seems like a long time, but it is more a beginning than an end. This is like a graduating doctor who makes choices about specialisation and how to choose further training. Acupuncture currently lacks postgraduate *sensory* training, so for graduates there is an issue as to how best to develop sensory skills. Western doctors have multiple, organised, long-term possibilities to develop their skills; acupuncturists do not – at least with respect to their Five Element diagnoses.

The power of habit formation

Diagnosing CFs is your main job. Developing the right habits means you improve more quickly and become more consistent sooner rather than later. Great performances in any field depend upon sufficient practise. Of course, an important degree of expertise comes just by being in practice, but the essential skills for diagnosing CFs improve much faster if you also practise *outside* the treatment room. Why? Observation and performance skills – diagnosing the patient's colour, odour, sound and emotion – need to become everyday habits.

James Clear has written a book on **habit formation**.[4] Let me summarise some of his thoughts. Find what works for you.

1 Take an automatic habit, such as something you do first thing upon waking in the morning and notice a sequence of four or five steps. These are ones that will not require special effort; you just do them, unconsciously. What are they? For me? 'Hear the alarm, find it and turn it off, relax back into bed, tell myself I should get up, feel my body for willingness', and so on.

2 Create an intention/idea for two or three new habits, for example, whilst greeting a patient I will scan the face for colour (or the vitality of the spirit), fluctuating back and forth. Wonder if this is too big, or too much to do alongside greeting the patient and maybe reduce it to scanning only for colour at one location. Another suggestion: just as I re-enter the room after stepping out while the patient changes into a gown, I sniff for an odour and label it the best I can.

3 James Clear suggests you make any habit (in your case to do with sensing colour, odour, sound or emotion) ridiculously small at first – so you cannot fail to complete it.

4 Ridiculously small will be different for different people. Specify when, what and where. For example: 'When I first greet the patient' (when), I will observe for the colour, lateral to the eyes' (what), 'wherever I first meet him/her' (where). Or, in the same context (maybe easier because of eye contact), 'I will notice the eyes to assess the spirit'. Design this to suit however you work: just keep it small and simple. Make it hard to fail. You can add more later. This is an important starting principle.

5 For memory and recording's sake, it is useful to think how to rate and record the vitality of the spirit. For example, using a scale of 1 to 5, where 1 is spirit is diminished and 5 is spirit is radiant.

The next step after the first habit is in place is to do what Clear calls **habit stacking**, that is, attaching another small habit to the first, so you are building a sequence or chain of habits all focused on diagnosis. For example, you could follow the first habit with expressing joy at seeing them and noting their response (basically a Fire test: see Chapter 8, page 59). Or, if you shake hands, you could rate the hand temperature from 1 (cold) to 5 (hot).

An important concern is not to add in something as large as 'test Water', unless you have already integrated the 'parts' of testing Water, which is more complex than testing Fire (see Chapter 11, Testing Water, page 87).

However, even testing Fire may be too complicated if you haven't learned how to express joy on demand. Normally, our emotions happen to us. We *find* ourselves sad, angry, hurt or whatever. But we can also *decide* to enter into joy, anger, respect, fear, and so on. There is an important difference between being subject to an emotion and deliberately expressing an emotion. So, another early skill to develop might be: 'Learn to express joy on demand'.

If you can't express joy on demand, then learn to do that first (Chapter 8, page 59). In Chapters 8 to 12 there are many suggestions of the mini skills to develop for each of the Five Elements.

Once you have decided what to practise (keep it small), work both on your own, but also with others. *Comparisons with others are like gold dust.* It could be anyone who is interested, but obviously your classmates or fellow graduates are the ideal practise mates.

Another Clear principle is to **connect practise with pleasure**. Make deals with yourself to only do something pleasurable – like chit-chatting with a friend or reading a newspaper with a cup of tea, when you have practised a specific exercise for X minutes. That is, reward yourself for practising.

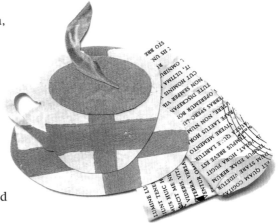

With any exercise you do, think about what you learned (however small) and celebrate it. Reward yourself with whatever feels good. What is rewarded gets repeated.

Clear recommends tracking your progress, that is, have some sort of journal where you **record any effort made** and what you learned, however small. Seeing what you have done can be a strong motivator. Ideally, tracking should be a motivator and if not, don't do it. I am not sure how quickly you can apply these principles, but I know you will benefit.

In Chapter 2, we look at developing rapport, an issue that JR Worsley said was important, but about which he said very little.

2

Building and maintaining rapport

'Rapport is the ability to enter someone else's world, to make them feel that you understand them, and that you have a common bond.'

Tony Robbins

The first stage of testing: building rapport

Rapport is the first stage of emotion testing; it lubricates the whole process of diagnosis and treatment. Rapport is created when people become psychologically closer. 'Closer' means that what they have in common becomes foreground, not so much consciously, but nevertheless felt, as if we thought, 'I just feel comfortable with this person. I'm not sure why.'.

I appreciate that two questions can arise in some practitioners' minds:
1 Do I want to do this at all – why can't I just be myself?
2 If I match and become like the other, will I lose myself?

The answer to the first question is that we match incessantly and mainly unconsciously; otherwise we couldn't care for our children, know how our friends feel, or watch a film with any emotional understanding. The answer to the second question is 'Yes, you can lose yourself' and that issue, which could include 'picking up' the patient's symptoms, is an important part of this chapter. For now, I would say that deliberate, conscious matching does not result in picking up symptoms. But we will return to this issue.

First of all, what not to do. People often want to differentiate themselves from others by being smarter, faster or more successful: note the excitement around the Olympics. Such an attitude has no place in the treatment room.

Rapport created by focusing on our similarities, has benefits. Patients with whom you have excellent rapport will:

- give information more readily
- relax and be available for your emotion tests
- put one hundred percent of themselves on the couch, making it easier for their energy to change
- be more likely to evaluate treatment positively
- stay with treatment longer, and
- be more likely to recommend you to others.

Rapport is worth developing. It is generated in three basic ways.

1 At the beginning, **by giving useful/necessary information** about the whole process of treatment to put patients at ease and maybe elicit some 'Why?' questions, which again are opportunities to build more rapport. Your patient's last visit might have been to the doctor so they will notice that you are different.

2 By **noticing where you and the patient have things in common that overlap and drawing them out**. This is done verbally, eliciting what is current in the patient's life and matching it **from** yours. People feel more comfortable with people like themselves!

3 By **non-verbal matching**, where you become more like your patient non-verbally: for example, what speed your bodies move, how fast you think and how fast you talk. Patients need not notice that you are matching them; they can feel comfortable because they are with someone who is like them.

Giving useful/necessary information

For many people acupuncture will be new. Or maybe they had some from the chiropractor or osteopath or some other alternative practitioner. Patients need to know how long your first appointment is, and the array of questions you will be asking. For example, 'I've come for my painful knee. Why are you asking about my bowels, perspiration, sleep, and so on?'.

Find out what they know, correct misapprehensions and fill in gaps. Imagine *you* are going for acupuncture for the first time and have no idea how the process goes. Do you work in someone else's clinic or at home or in a clinic with other acupuncturists? Is this someone you know or someone you have never seen before? Some things patients need to know may come from your website. You may have sent the person a leaflet before they meet you. What questions does it answer? Did they read it? These issues will be individual to your practice.

Anticipate the questions a new patient will have; answer them in whatever way you can, for example, a leaflet, over the phone or when you first meet them. And then check: 'Do you have any other questions before we begin?'.

Overlaps (what we have in common) and drawing them out

An important habit to develop when you meet someone new is to notice how *different* you are or how *similar* you are? With patients, focus on how similar you are. Overlaps are what we have in common – like having children, playing a sport, going to a night class, having lost a child, or having been to Las Vegas. Just looking at someone for the first time is a poor guide to knowing a person, simply because so much of what is important to us is not obvious from the outside.[5] We build rapport by focusing on similarities.

In a new class, I asked for a volunteer who thought that he or she was most different from me. A lady in her 50s responded, and I asked her to tell me something about herself. She immediately began to describe her family and how two of her children had been very ill and what a struggle it was for her. After a few minutes, I told her about my daughter's severe health condition from birth. Soon, we were both exchanging information about some of the most important moments in our lives. We both were in tears and ended up hugging.

In a group held in Bristol many years ago, a 5'1", female practitioner described a patient who she found difficult. He was a 6'2" biker whose leathers and boots left grease on the couch. She insisted that they had nothing in common – nothing that could lead to any sense of rapport. When she came to the following session, she said she had some feedback. She asked the biker what it was about his biker's gear that he liked so much. He explained that he loved riding with his mates, wearing his gear and parading through town 'looking good'.

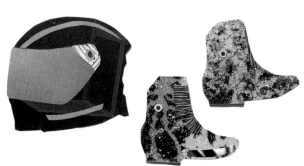

She had just bought a new party dress to wear at the weekend. She described to him shopping, finding this dress and buying it. She'd tried it on, loved it and had already showed it to a friend. The biker smiled and said something along the lines of: 'Yeh, it's great looking good, isn't it?'. And he described again riding through town on his bike.

Different genders, different contexts, but what lay underneath was similar if not the same. She reported one more thing. After treatment, he got up, scrunched up the paper towel and wiped some grease off the couch, apologised for the grease and thanked her for the treatment. That had not happened before. A brief focus on similarity made a difference. Technically, this is called **chunking up** and is described in more detail in the appendix on advanced rapport-building skills, page 115.

Try it out Whenever you notice someone doing or talking about something which you don't like, before you dismiss it, **chunk up** by asking:
- 'What do you like about it?'
- 'What does it do for you?', or
- 'What is important to you about it?'

A practitioner from Wales described a patient. He was Asian and he endlessly complained that his family was not accepted in the community. He admitted he expressed it by grumbling. Later he explained how important 'family/community' was to him and how much it upset him because he wanted to be 'part of the community'. The practitioner immediately understood how important community was to her too. When this was acknowledged, closer rapport followed. Chunking up is a direct path to what we have in common.

To summarise, a core question is: 'What is important about X, where X is something that the person invests time/attention in'? This can be varied to suit the context, by varying the words:
- What is it about X that you enjoy?
- You really enjoy that. What matters to you about that?
- Why is X important to you?

To chunk up, find words that work for you. Discover higher-level similarities.

Non-verbal matching

Non-verbal matching has two purposes and an added benefit. Its **first purpose** is to **develop rapport, gain agreement and enhance cooperation**. For example, matching body posture can make the patient more comfortable and thus more receptive.

Its **second purpose** is, by being like the patient, to **further your diagnosis**. Matching the patient's posture more exactly can begin to produce diagnostic information, for example, about the patient's constricted chest and the flow or lack of flow of energy in the body. This type of matching is diagnostic but requires care that the practitioner does not 'pick up' symptoms. More about that later.

Taking matching seriously requires time and effort. Matching involves deliberate observation and a degree of behavioural flexibility. It not only takes time to develop, but for some, who may feel that their identity is at stake, it needs to proceed slowly, so they are convinced that they can match consciously and not lose themselves. When you match, match deliberately and consciously.

Supreme flexibility to build rapport I remember a young, female student with her first patient, carrying out the traditional diagnosis. As her supervisor, I entered the room a bit late and found the patient striding back and forth and talking ten to the dozen. The student practitioner was standing in the corner, moving a step or two in either direction, pad in hand. I explained who I was and asked him to sit. He said he preferred to stand so he walked and I also conducted my examination moving as space allowed. I decided that he was a Fire CF with Phlegm Misting the Heart. I left the room. To my delight, when I later asked the practitioner about her diagnosis, she said, having done her examination standing and walking, that he was a Fire CF with Phlegm Misting the Heart. Quality matching!

To be clear about the actual use of matching, we need to briefly discuss **mirror-neurons**. These are neurons in the brain/nervous system that fire both when someone acts and when someone observes an action performed by another. These neurons were discovered by an Italian scientist who had the brains of two monkeys wired up. He noticed that, when one monkey was eating a banana, a specific part of his brain was engaged, and the *same* part of an observing monkey's brain was also engaged, indicating this was the way the second monkey knew what the first monkey was doing.

We take this awareness for granted. Mirror neurons are the basis of our ability to imitate and learn from others – leading to ordinary skills like learning to walk, knowing what others are feeling or learning to talk. They are the basis of an important learning principle: 'Monkey see, monkey do'. In the process of evolution, the entry of mirror neurons was cosmic: it changed how fast some animals could learn and evolve.

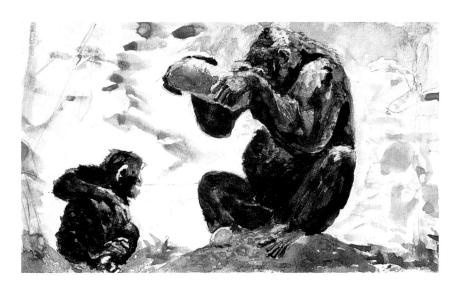

Mirror neurons are illustrated by a chimpanzee who observes its mother cracking a nut with a rock and then tries to imitate her by doing the same. So, mirror neurons confer upon a species an ability to learn from each other through imitation. Imitation accounts for the great success of humans in the process of evolution. Scratching, yawning and stretching are often mediated by mirror neurons. Without mirror neurons, we would be blind to the actions, intentions and emotions of other people.

A useful introduction to mirror neurons is a ten-minute TEDTalk video on YouTube called 'The neurons that shaped civilization', where VS Ramachandran, a neuroscientist, explains what mirror neurons are and why they are important.[6] Mirror neurons have made empathy and imitation possible and made humans top of the evolutionary tree.[7]

The purpose and dangers of matching

Matching has two purposes:

1 To **develop rapport** and achieve all the benefits which good rapport can bring
2 To **understand the patient** by being like them, thus improving your diagnosis and, possibly, getting the CF

However, **matching states** has a drawback: ask yourself if you are a natural and unconscious matcher. If you are, you may easily feel what others are feeling, you can remember being with someone in a negative state and later not feeling so good yourself. In addition, there are incidents, TV shows, films which you know will upset you and you avoid them. *If so, pay careful attention to the following table.*

Make a distinction between a positive state and a negative one – one where you feel good and one where you feel bad. Matching others' good states is fine: people often rely on others to get through difficult times and we all have some experience of having our internal state being affected positively by others. However, in general:

Matching	Positive states	Negative states
Consciously – deliberately, with awareness	OK	With care
Unconsciously – instinctively, without awareness	OK	Not good

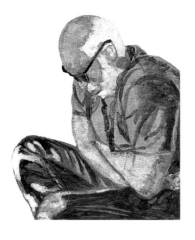

When I say matching a state, matching posture is in effect a way of matching a state. As an example, in a group practice session, I was sitting out, but was observing another participant. He was slouching and when I achieved a similar posture and my mind focused on him, I then felt that his Heart dropped downwards (I would call it **Heart-sink**) and the same thing happened to me. I was now no longer in a good state; the feeling scared me and I straightened up abruptly to change state. I had experienced the other person's drop into sadness.

I learned to take care not to *unconsciously* match others' **unresourceful states**, for example, depression, restlessness or anger. When unconsciously matching another's negative state, we can take on something which worsens our health for no one's benefit. Do practitioners do this? I believe so. If you work with unwell people, it is hard, sometimes, *not* to do it. Matching is a double-edged sword.

In a class of 25, there are often three or four students who, at the beginning of the course, are already aware that they might 'pick up something' from close contact and unconscious matching of another person. This is my informal deduction, gleaned from asking classes when matching is introduced. There are others who find out later that they are 'unconscious matchers' and can 'take on' unresourceful states.

And there are others who never experience unconscious matching, and thus think it is nonsense.

So, how is it best to proceed with matching?
• Learn how to match consciously
• Become aware of how often you unconsciously match (for example, loved ones, family, fictional characters)
• Learn to match negative states, but only consciously
• Be aware when not to match
• Notice whether, during matching, you have taken on an unresourceful state

So, with care, let us start with what it might be useful to match.

What you might match

Some matching done well is much better than a lot done badly. First, consider the options and later we will discuss your best choices: for now, remember that good matching can create strong rapport. You could match:
• the **tempo** of speech, body movement, thinking
• a repetitive **body posture/gesture**
• the patient's **voice as resonating with the Elements** (laughing, singing, weeping, groaning and shouting)
• the patient's **breathing pattern**
• **key/repetitive gestures** (timing is important)
• **key words/phrases** used by the patient (timing is important)
• **sensory predicates** (a person's use of words).

Some of the above can be matched **directly**, as opposed to **indirectly**. For example, you might adjust your tempo to be slower because the patient is overall slower than you. You speak at 70 mph; they speak at 40 mph and so you slow down. I would call that direct. However, if you take a gesture like hiking your glasses back up your nose with your index finger – something that recurs every three or four minutes – then this needs to be 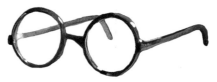 done indirectly, that is, by incorporating it into your behaviour as if it is normal for you and not in any way directly mimicking the patient. You do it not as an immediate response but, as it were, naturally, as part of your behaviour. Take care to distinguish direct and indirect matching.[8]

Let's look at the matching options in more detail:

Matching	Direct	Adjusting	Examples
*Matchings that **don't** require timing*			
Tempo of: • speech • movement • thinking	Adjust to patient's tempo in three ways, one at a time. Speech/thinking will be close	Easier to slow than speed up. Can be frustrating and hard to do	Very slow speech; agitated movements; a mind which makes quick leaps
Posture	Become closer to patient's posture	Forwards/ backwards; erect/slumped	Degrees of accuracy from gross to subtle
Voice	Five Element sound becomes closer to that of patient's	Based on Five Element sounds	An Earth CF practitioner puts 'shout' into their voice
Breathing	Match rate and area (chest, Middle, or Lower Burner)	Can be quite exact	Easiest done when holding a hand – just after/whilst pulse taking
*Matchings that **do** require timing*			
Key gestures *See page 117*	**Indirect** 'Integrated into' practitioner's behaviour at appropriate moments	Often the arms/ hands/face	Cutting with edge of hand; palms upwards with eyes wide open
Key words *See page 117*	'Fitted into' what practitioner says	Both word(s) and tone	Spoken as if it's my word. May accompany gestures
Sensory predicates *See page 121*	Notice visual/auditory/ tactile/kinaesthetic words/bias and take these on yourself	You need the flexibility/practise to do this	Patient talks mainly about what they see and practitioner then matches

I would suggest that the first three, **tempo**, **posture** and **voice** are basic and, for most practitioners, sufficient. So, let us look at these more closely.

Matching tempo

Tempo covers speech, body movements and thinking. Start by making a comparison between the speed/rate of your speech and that of the patient. Is their rate faster, slower or the same? If it's the same, ignore it. If it's faster or slower, can you adjust it by becoming more like them – not necessarily the same as them, but closer?

Don't just practise in class, but elsewhere – watching TV, listening to the radio or with friends/acquaintances. Ask yourself: 'Am I slower or faster or the same?'. Then adjust. By doing this with several people – classmates, friends, people in shops – you will gradually become aware of speech tempo and how to adjust to it. That is the goal.

Then do the same with movement and thinking using the same process. (Matching a slow thinker who thinks out loud can initially be tortuous.) Compare yourself to the other person and, if there is a difference, adjust. Gradually, you will be able to do this without effort.

Matching posture

This mainly applies when you are sitting with a patient. It comes down to leaning forwards/backwards, legs open/closed, slumped/upright. Becoming similar in posture requires observation, thought, adjustment and maintaining or changing as the patient changes. This can be practised anywhere, for example, in class or in a café. It simply requires noticing and adapting, noticing and more adapting – until you are aware that something has clicked.

Matching voice

Sounds and the content of the voice are processed by different parts of the brain. It is not necessarily easy to listen to both simultaneously. We *hear* the content; we tend to be *affected* by the sound. With patients, our tendency is to listen to content, for fear that we miss what the patient is saying. However, practitioners need to learn to listen to sound and this is best done by listening to voices, recorded or otherwise, where there is no obligation to hear content, for example, watching TV, radio, recordings or eavesdropping (more on this in Chapter 5, page 33).

As you learn to label the sounds, it is useful to imitate the sounds yourself. This is not necessarily easy. You may be a Metal CF and hear the 'sing' in another's voice and when you try it, it comes out as a pale imitation, hardly rising and falling at all, and you then know what you need to practise to achieve more flexibility. Practise will make matching possible and accurate matching can develop your state and you will hear better. This match increases your flexibility and your ability to read the sounds in the voice.

Work at and become proficient in the matchings discussed so far and you will establish 'good enough' rapport.

Summary for rapport

Advanced matching skills If you have the time and head space to explore other kinds of matching skills, take a look at the appendix, 'Advanced rapport-building skills', page 115. Also in that section you will find descriptions of useful techniques drawn from neuro-linguistic programming (NLP), which has long been a strong influence on my practice. All of these advanced skills will enrich your ability to understand your patients, and repay the effort it takes to assimilate and absorb them.

- **Strong rapport** can be achieved by matching and there are many ways to match.
- Care must be taken with unconscious matching to **avoid taking on negative states**.
- Experiment, but in the end choosing **a few simple ways of matching and developing the specific skills** is probably best and is probably what most practitioners can manage, at least when training.
- **Tempo**, **posture** and **overlaps** are probably the three basic ways of matching.
- Matching can also be **diagnostic** but this requires a higher degree of matching skill.

3
Colour on the face

Five Element facial colours

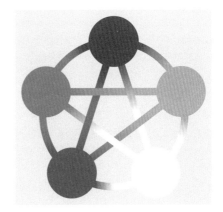

Element	Colour
Fire	Red
Earth	Yellow
Metal	White
Water	Blue
Wood	Green

With colour we have a vocabulary translated from Chinese. The Element colours look fine displayed on a chart, but actual facial colours, to put it mildly, are somewhat different. **Red** for the Fire Element often becomes in practice **lack of red**, not a shiny lack of red, but often a paleness and sometimes a pale-dull colour. **Blue** ranges between a light blue and black. For Earth it depends on what you think **yellow** is: canary yellow, ochre, burnt sienna, the literal colour of a handful of earth, when it is wet or damp or dry. So, with no standardised colour chart, it is inevitable to defer to an experienced clinical supervisor with previous experience of colour and successful diagnosis. But how does the supervisor learn, and do supervisors agree? Why worry? I don't know, but I did.[9]

Location on the face

The Five Element colours are located on the face in the following places:
- lateral to the eyes
- under the eyes
- in the laugh lines (nasolabial folds), and
- around the mouth.

First, train yourself to look, in sequence, from one location to the next. It's a basic habit and requires practise. It may be difficult at the first moment of contact, but once you are chatting, colour observation is easier. When lighting conditions are poor, however, it might be best to ask the patient to approach a window or even step outside to find the best light.[10]

What about the actual colour? There is no colour chart, but often, through careful examination, we can eliminate three Element colours and end up with two, for example, maybe yellow, maybe green. Or, we can exclude yellow, green and blue and wonder whether it is white or lack of red (that is, pale). The learning process is irregular and requires attention and then more and more attention. It is best shared with others, observing over and over again, until it becomes automatic and has a wider sensory base.

This is paradoxical, but sometimes a colour gets resolved not by observing colour, but, for example, treatment on Earth works so the colour *must* be an Earth one and therefore is yellow: definitely circular reasoning and faulty as the four indicators are meant to be independent. Or, a clinical supervisor points at a patient's colour and, with authority, labels it yellow, or 'an Earth colour', and the student has valuable feedback. It may be an unreasonable goal early on to master colour. The actual amount of feedback varies and, in a year-long clinical, developing certainty may not be a reasonable goal. Therefore, the learning/practise process needs to be maintained by the graduate once in practice.

So, how else to proceed? One way is to verify the CF by other means, for example symptom change, the patient feeling 'better in her/himself' and on that basis say: 'Yes, what we are looking at is probably yellow, the colour of Earth, because treatment on Earth has worked'. Or, take a walk on a busy street and just notice different facial colours and then label them if you can – at first, go for volume, and observe lots of people, rather than accuracy.

The next step is to develop a *range* of colour that will be manifested by Earth CFs as we don't expect there to be only one shade of the Earth colour, but a variety with more or less Damp, more or less Heat. Bear in mind that there are 5,000 ethnic groups with varying skin colours and on the Five Element posters, only one Earth colour. This suggests lots of rigorous, sensory comparisons, checks with others and an attitude of ongoing flexibility and practise – in the clinic, observing with others and observing in daily life. Colour observation has many approaches and is a lifelong task.

This is not the most welcome conclusion, but the most practical whether you are a student or practitioner.

Three ways to develop sensitivity to colour

1 The first is to **observe known CFs** and learn from verified examples. A good opportunity is what are called 'CF days' when up to 50+ practitioners who know their CFs gather and sit in CF groups and talk about how they know they are a specific CF.

2 A second useful way is to **compare the colour of at least two or more people at the same moment** and look rapidly back and forth. If they are fellow students, they can be asked to bring their faces close together and in good light. If in public, the observation will have to be alternating, back and forth. The task is to notice both similarities, and differences. If you know CFs of the people being observed, so much the better.

3 A third way, which develops a memory bank, is **in daily life to observe the colour of whoever you meet**. You can't do this all day every day, of course, but you can spend some time regularly just looking at colour. At first you look at the relevant areas just for colour in general, and then, as soon as you 'see' the colour you label it, using your own colour words which in turn you begin to associate with an Element. For example: 'It's a shiny, glossy, pale bluey-white and it might be Metal, it might be Water'. You can do this on the street, in cafés, at a leisure centre – wherever people congregate. Ideally, this is best done with a study buddy.[11]

4
Odour

Five Element odours

Element	Odour
Fire	Scorched
Earth	Fragrant
Metal	Rotten
Water	Putrid
Wood	Rancid

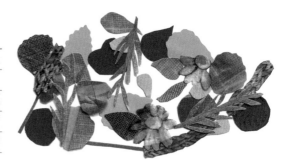

Earlier, I described JR Worsley picking up a patient's smell from a distance. If you don't already notice odours easily, and most people don't, there are some ways to improve your ability to smell. It is best to make these exercises enjoyable. Involve others if you can and feel better simply because resurrecting an unused sense is a good thing to do. More importantly, a clear odour can confirm a CF and simplify the whole process.

I would suggest there are three stages:

1 Consciously noticing more smells
2 Labelling the smells the best you can
3 Learning to use Five Element labels

Some suggestions for noticing odours

- When a patient enters the treatment room, ask them to change into a gown and leave them for a few minutes. There are two important moments. One is **when you re-enter the treatment room**, before you say anything to the patient. We habituate quickly to odours. The other is when you **remove a blanket** from the prone patient to carry out the

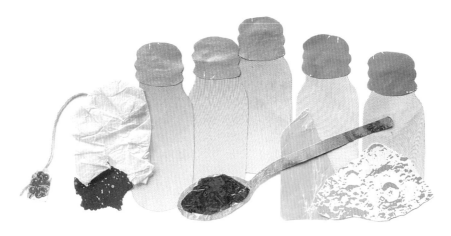

physical exam, in the first few seconds – close enough to 'catch' an odour. Give yourself the best opportunities.

- **Find odours which seem to typify the Element**. For example, where you go: 'Oh, so that is scorched', (or fragrant, rotten, putrid or rancid), then attempt to bottle that smell (see point 5 below) so you have a model odour for a particular Element odour. A public urinal or ammonia might smell 'putrid'; an ironing board might smell 'scorched'; rotting leaves might smell 'rotten'; olive oil gone off might smell 'rancid'; and dried-out flowers might smell 'fragrant'.[12]

- **You may need to change your attitude to smelling**. People nowadays avoid what were once ordinary and significant odours and cover them up with a more acceptable, 'nice' odours. There is the need to ask your patient to come, at least once, with no added odours, that is, cosmetics, perfumes, shaving gel, etc. They may resist, but you can insist.

- **Condition yourself to notice odours** as you move from one room to another or from inside a building to outside or vice versa. This is not difficult to do, although you need to persist for several days – maybe 20 – for the habit to become fixed. Any transition from one contained area to the next is an opportunity. I once had a cat and that is what she seemed to do. She would wait inside the cat door and sniff before deciding whether to go out or remain inside.

- **Get some 'smell bottles'**, opaque, smallish containers. Number them on the bottom, 1 to 4 or 1 to 5 and put into them different smelling substances – some jam, coffee, tea (various types), dried leaves or petals of a flower, a piece of cheese (various types), some underarm hair, shaving soap, olive oil, perfumes (various types), a piece of fish (cooked or not), a small piece of scorched cloth from the ironing board, or rotting meat. With the tops on, and numbers out of sight, mix the bottles so you don't know which is which. Pick one, take the top off with eyes closed and sniff. Identify the source or if not, describe the smell as best you can. Describing in your own words starts you developing a 'smell' vocabulary. Replace the top and carry on. If you can correctly label them all, change the substances and start again. If you can't, practise till you can. Then change one or two or all substances and repeat. Some deliberate smelling every day helps to develop the habit.

- **If you are not a 'hugger'**, take a risk and hug a few friends when you first meet them. Snuggle your nose into their neck and sniff. With fellow students or practitioners, where you both know the purpose, this is easy. Do your best to label the smell, even if it is likely to be soap, perfume, or various cosmetics.

Odour can be important. For most of us, getting skilled at discerning odour requires some effort, but the rewards are clear.

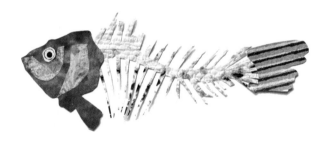

5
Sound in the voice

Five Element voice sounds

Element	Sound
Fire	Laugh
Earth	Sing
Metal	Weep
Water	Groan
Wood	Shout

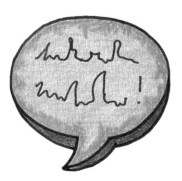

Representing these voice sounds visually may help some people – a transfer from ear to eye.

Laugh

The label 'laugh' does not mean an actual laugh, but it is close. The voice goes up in pitch as it does when we literally laugh, but not so quickly. So, a voice resonating with Fire will not be an actual laugh but will resemble it in that it will contain slower-paced rises in pitch.

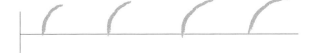

Sing

A voice that 'sings' will go up and down in pitch leading us to call it 'sing-songy', or lullaby-like. By contrast, the laughing voice just goes up.

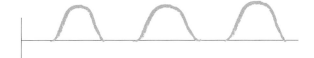

Weep

Whereas the laugh goes up and up and up and the sing goes up and down and up and down, the weeping voice goes maybe up a little but then down and repeatedly drops off as if its power runs out, recovers and then runs out again – mainly in volume. It is as if the machine producing the sound is tired and running out of energy.

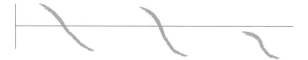

Groan

A groan in a voice neither goes up nor down, but stays level, almost as if not to disturb the dangerous snake last seen under the bed.

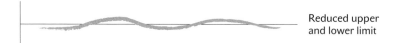

Reduced upper and lower limit

Shout

A shout contains words with a volume emphasis on one syllable, as in: 'I did **not** say **that** to her; I am r**eal**ly up**set**'. The whole speech may be short or long, even quiet or loud, but periodically within it there are syllables which are given distinctly more emphasis than the others. Say the sentence in quotes above and emphasise the words shown in **bold**. Do this first with whole sentence relatively loud; then say the sentence relatively quietly, but still with the emphasis on the words in bold. A shout is emphasis or *relative* and *abrupt* loudness.

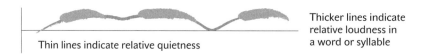

Thin lines indicate relative quietness

Thicker lines indicate relative loudness in a word or syllable

Another possibility is that there is an absence of 'shout' in the voice. This occurs when we judge that the person is or should be angry (there is an abuse, an abuser and wrongness), but there is no evidence or show of anger. The emphasis which we label a 'shout' is absent.

A difference with sound

Unlike colour and odour, which before treatment will probably remain constant, sound is more complex and changeable.

Sound by its nature will vary more than colour or odour, depending on the context created by the practitioner. By context, I mean the emotional context they create. If the practitioner 'tests' (see Chapters 8 to 12 on testing the Elements) or 'generates' a context for joy, sympathy, respect, fear and anger, then the voice will not be as constant as with colour or odour. For example, a Water CF can be appropriately angry and shout. Or, a Fire CF may occasionally be angry and shout. Or, a Metal CF can express sympathy and sing (a little). There is more variation than with colour and odour. So, assessing sound can be more complex.

Being sure about sound has an extra challenge for the practitioner. One strategy is to test emotions and whilst doing so take small diversions into listening for the current sound.

When the sound doesn't resonate with the emotion, you have a strong clue from two Elements as to the CF. For example, when we observe a patient whose emotion is anger (from the face) and at the same time whose sound is groaning (from the voice). We notice the incongruity. These could indicate the person is either a Wood CF or a Water CF. Equally, we might observe a patient saying in a flat, monotone voice (a groan): 'I am happy; really, I am'. Which one do we trust; the sound or what the patient says? It can be tricky to separate the two.

So, it is important to learn to recognise the sounds in the voice independently of any connection with emotions. How to do this?

First, we need to **separate the two modes of listening**. One is listening to words – what people are saying – as we do when taking notes, and the other is listening to sound – as we do when closing our eyes and listening to music, particularly instrumental music. They are different and use different parts of the brain. This makes it difficult initially to do both at the same time, although I believe that musicians and singers have already learned to hear sounds and words together. Put some background music on and have a conversation which requires careful attention to what is being said. You can switch rapidly back and forth, but listening consciously to both simultaneously does not happen easily.

When listening to **content** we might:
- lean forwards
- look more intensely at the speaker
- maybe put one ear forwards
- consider what to write down
- repeat the words or make notes.

When listening for **sound** we might:
- close our eyes or defocus, go inside
- let the sound 'come to me'
- relax more.

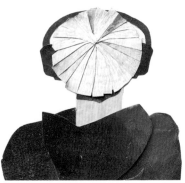

Watch someone listening to music through headphones, and observe their body language.

So, it is necessary to become skilful at listening for sound when another person is talking. An important first step is to differentiate listening to sound and listening to content, so that the ability to switch is clearly under your control. You can achieve this by being under no pressure to hear the content and then switch back and forth, listen for 20 seconds to sound, 20 seconds to content and so on. You can use:
- recordings of patients
- people speaking on TV or the radio
- people in a group who have no obligation/need to listen to content.

This 'switching' can also be done in a group exercise where two people talk and others switch back and forth from listening to sounds to listening to content every ten to 20 seconds. The interval should not be too long as you are developing a 'sense' of each so that you can later be able to *consciously* make the switch. You can also do this in a variety of contexts, including eavesdropping in a café.

A **second step** is to **listen to sound when under no pressure to be hearing content** and while you do this to begin to label the sounds in the voice: laugh, sing, weep, groan and shout. If you practise in a group, have two people chatting, while the rest listen to sound and ask: 'Who has more shout, sing, weep, and so on? or simply: 'What is the sound in this voice now?'. The talkers can be asked to speak about different subjects, for example, anything they are angry about, pleased about, fearful of and listeners can listen for changes in the sound. You can develop practices that work for you.

Without such practise, practitioners can get stuck in listening to content and never become skilful at finding the most inappropriate sound. Can you label the predominant sound in the voice of your parents or friends? My mother was a Wood CF and when I was young I had practise listening to a 'shout': it was scary and, of course, I didn't know how to label it at the time.

A **third step** is to **do exercises whereby you are clear about the differences between one sound and another**. A useful exercise is the following: **A** and **B** talk. **A** has been instructed to be angry and **B** has been instructed to be fearful. Switch roles and emotions.

People listen to speech about five plus times faster than they speak: in the time it takes a speaker to say 100 words, the listener has the capacity 'to hear' 500+ words.[13] This means that while the patient is talking, the practitioner requires only a part of their capacity for attention to hear the content. So, there are options.

If you want to hear the sound, it will be best not to notice colour or odour at the same time. It will be best *not* to be writing down what is said. Instead, observe the accompanying emotion and *judge the resonance*. Resonance is defined as: what sound fits with what emotion, that is, a laugh goes with joy, a sing goes with sympathy, and so on.

In the end, being adept at hearing sound requires learning to shift back and forth rapidly. Even if you are losing a little content, it is worth it if you are hearing and labelling the predominant sound.

Summary for evaluating sound

- At first **listen to sounds separately**. Find a way where you have no responsibility for getting the content. For example, watch TV and just listen to the newscaster's voice for sounds, not content, and hear the predominant sound. Enjoy this. Do it while watching the news and share your perceptions with others. I am pretty sure I know the 'sound in the voice' of most newscasters and the PM and several cabinet ministers. Use recorded conversations or radio in the same way. Unfortunately, there is no way to verify the sound, but it is good practice for knowing how to just listen for sound.

- Then, attempt to **listen to the words only** and record exactly what was said.

- Only then, **flip back and forth** between sound and content, say every ten or 20 seconds and gain control of what you are paying attention to – sound or content.

- Then **listen to sound** and **watch the face for emotion**, and ask: 'Do these resonate or don't they?'. If they resonate and both fit the context, that is probably not the CF. If they don't, persist with other sounds and a sound/emotion disconnect will become clearer.

- Think of times where you would feel joy, sympathy, grief, fear and anger and work up some feeling. Whilst still feeling, **speak in the best 'resonating' voice**. Judge yourself and repeat to get the voice even more 'in synch'.

Sound is important, not just when you are diagnosing, but when you are testing emotions (see Chapters 8 to 12 for this). You need to be able to deliberately use each of the sounds. For instance, when testing anger you need to put a 'shout' in your voice. For example: '**What**, she said **that** to you?'. So, as well as hearing the sounds, acquiring the facility to express them is important.

> **Learning to use each of the five sounds** Work with a partner. Make five cards with the labels for sounds on them: shout, laugh, sing, weep and groan. On your own, or better, with a partner, shuffle the cards and then turn one over. Whatever the sound, for example, sing, talk with a sing in your voice for ten seconds. Repeat with the next card. A partner can feed back to you on which are your best voice sounds and which are your least good ones. Swap over. If one sound is particularly difficult, practise it on its own.

6

Four important aspects of emotions

Five Element emotions

Element	Emotions
Fire	Joy/sadness
Earth	Sympathy/worry/overthinking
Metal	Grief
Water	Fear
Wood	Anger

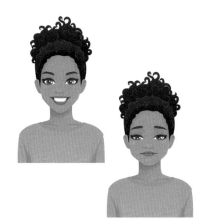

1 How do negative emotions cause disease?

When we experience an emotion, there is a habitual focus of attention. With anger, we focus on the 'abuser' or some idea of what is being done to us. The focus on the abuser may be either a direct sensory experience when the abuser is present or a mental image of the abuser when he/she is not present. With sadness we focus to some degree on body sensations but more on rejection, who disappointed us, or thoughts about: 'What's wrong with me?'. With worry we focus on our concerns. However, we represent them in our heads, for example, the increasing pain in our abdomen and what this could mean, or the person who was seen hanging around our front door. With grief we focus on the loss. We may visualise what we have lost or talk to ourselves about it. With fear we focus on an imagined violation that may happen in the future and how bad could it be. These foci of attention are usually in themselves harmful.

At the same time, we do *not* focus directly on our bodies and the accompanying, negative, bodily sensations. So, we do not fully experience them.[14] Were we to do so, we would respond differently to anger, sadness, worry, grief and fear. We would be more likely to do whatever we could to reduce the discomfort, just as when we hit our thumb with a hammer, we do whatever we can to soothe or reduce the pain. It is not that these sensations go *totally* unnoticed, but they seem less important than the external foci mentioned above. Although emotions are called the **Internal Causes of Disease** we often experience them with little or diminished bodily awareness. This explains why many internal practices, which encourage increased awareness of the body, tend to limit the duration of negative emotions. For example, meditation, *tai chi*, focusing and *qi gong* and many other internal practices increase internal bodily awareness, which in turn increases our awareness of the impact of negative emotions and encourages us to find ways of reducing them. I hasten to add that the above-mentioned disciplines are not all the same. But one thing they have in common is an increasing sensitivity to our body and therefore we become more aware of the bodily sensations associated with negative emotions.

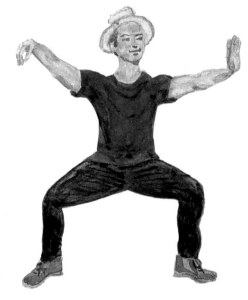

Take Wood, and its emotion, anger. I may, for example, be regularly angry at my neighbour who plays music late at night which, because of thin walls, I can't block it out, and it stops me from getting off to sleep. Ear plugs don't seem to make enough difference and, anyway, why should I have to wear earplugs in my own flat? The longer it happens, the more upset I get. I have spoken to the neighbour and been ignored. My mind focuses on the neighbour, the injustice or my rights. Would it not seem better to focus on what is effectively damaging me, that is, the bodily sensations that accompany my anger? Here are some of the sensations which accompany anger, taken from students in class who have deliberately remembered being angry and focused on their bodies – an unusual thing to do, but informative.

Wood: bodily sensations associated with feeling angry

Grinding teeth	Hardening of the eyes	Something flowing up the back of neck
Tension in the forehead	Eyes open and then tight	
Heat going to my head	Rising up feeling that drops after	Tight TMJ (temporomandibular or jaw) joints
Constriction in the throat		
Tunnel vision	Pain in the forehead	Head moving forwards
Breathing faster	Diaphragm pushing down on stomach	Nostrils opening
Conscious of heartbeat		Body trembling
Pressure around ears	Tightening of the jaw	Breath laboured and forced
Pressure in the chest	Stomach knotted up	Clenching fists
	Breath irregular	Burning sensation under rib cage
	Pounding in the heart	Eyes hurting

Many of these sensations are symptoms found in the TCM Liver or Gall Bladder syndromes. Others are clearly feelings of discomfort. To be convinced of the damage they do, stop, remember something you were/ are angry about, re-experience the moment of anger and pay attention to the accompanying bodily sensations. (If you can, do that now.) Most people find such an experience enlightening in that the bodily sensations accompanying anger (and every other negative emotion) are uncomfortable and diminish the healthy functioning of the body. The table above makes this obvious for Wood and it is equally true for the negative emotions associated with Fire (sadness), Earth (worry), Metal (grief) and Water (fear).

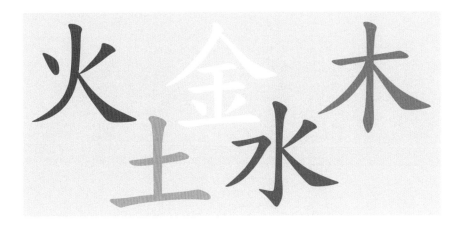

Below are some of the other bodily sensations that classes have reported when students have been asked to enter/remember some other Five Element negative emotions and then notice the accompanying bodily sensations.

Fire: bodily sensations associated with feeling sadness

Ache in chest	Body crumpling	Draining downward
Drop throat to stomach	Compression in chest	'Black' around heart
Face squeezed in and down	Heart feels crushed	As if knives stabbing chest
Dark and black in chest	Lips tense	Contracting inside
Eyes focus downward	Downward pressure on shoulders	Squeezing in upper body
Upper body collapsing		Stopped breathing
Hard to hold head up	Squeezing of eyes	Eyes look down
	Tears starting	

Earth: bodily sensations associated with worry/overthinking

Collapse in midriff	Faces muscles go slack	Head down, want to cry
Eye squinting, turning out	Collapsing in chest	Turning palms up
Almost lose balance	Squeezing into abdomen	Thoughts whirling
Eyes strained	Tightening across back	Hardly breathing in
Forehead furrowed	Head tilts or rolls	Arms tighten/withdraw
Occiput squeezed	Tight between shoulder blades	Bending in abdomen
Pressure down on neck		Arms/legs pull in
Back of neck squeezes	Hands tighten up	Want to collapse on floor

Metal: bodily sensations associated with grief

Abdominal slumping	Cheeks/face dropping	Breathing held
Chest pushed backwards	Tightness in chest	Restriction between shoulder blades
Head drops down	A pushing up with no strength	
Chest and into arms tight		Tight across back
Looking down at nothing	Contracting in chest	Gentle squeezing down
Wanting to collapse	Eyes feel tight/look down	Overall downward pressure
Gentle ache in chest area	Overall heaviness	Can't see out
	Palms up, neck forwards	

Water: bodily sensations associated with feeling fear

Tight in whole body	Body feels pulled backwards	Tight in chest
Eyes stressed and open		Squeezing in
Overall tight	Breath held	Like being strangled
Feeling nervy	Twitchy	Tightening in abdomen
Still	A draining downwards	Throat gets tight
Mouth open, jaw tight	Shoulders tight	Eyes get twitchy
	Feel rigid in middle of body	

None of these sensations are ones we want to experience on a regular basis. They are clearly part of the Internal Causes of Disease.

The participants who provided these examples had a mix of different CFs and only a proportion would be diagnosed with the CF associated with the emotion being experienced. What is significant is that each negative emotion has a typical array of negative sensations which when experienced repetitively, lead to some form of distress/illness.

You are reading about the experience of others. Ideally, it is best to do the exercises yourself. That is, remember a time when you experienced sadness, worry, grief, fear or anger. Let the bodily sensations rise and escalate. By *consciously* noticing the bodily sensations, the emotions won't take you over, as they might in real life. Keep paying attention to the bodily sensations and record them. These exercises will help to convince you that these sensations are the Internal Causes of Disease. The exercises are more easily done in a group.[15]

This approach – paying attention to sensations when dealing with one's own negative emotions – is supported by Professor Paul Ekman in a discussion hosted by the Dalai Lama and attended by some of the world's most sophisticated Buddhist meditators and some of the West's most respected scientists. And, maybe more importantly, it helps explain both the simplicity and positive effect of Five Element acupuncture and the Internal Causes of Disease.[16]

As a suggestion, if you know what your CF is, next time you experience a negative emotion, stop (yes, difficult) and focus exclusively on your sensations. What does that do?

For me, this calls into question the emotions recorded in English on some Five Element acupuncture charts, that is, joy/worry/grief/fear/anger or joy/sympathy/grief/fear/anger. In the first, joy is generally thought to be a positive emotion, although we can talk about 'excess joy' as a negative experience, but the chart says joy. In the second, sympathy also sounds positive compared to grief, fear or anger. I will address this issue in each Element chapter.

2 As an emotion tester, we also have a CF: how does that affect us?

The emotion resonating with our own CF, unlike colour, sound and odour, will impact how we understand or fail to understand others' emotions. By having a CF, we have an inbuilt bias.

Different people develop values according to their personal circumstances *and* in relation to their different CFs. For example, Fire and Water CFs may value interpersonal sincerity as it builds trust, but for slightly different reasons. The Fire CF, for example, will feel hurt at any dishonesty or betrayal; whereas the Water CF may feel fear or distrust at any dishonesty and resolve never to trust that person again. The external behaviour may seem similar. At the same time Fire CFs may value 'having fun or enjoyment' whereas the Water CF may put a relatively low value on fun.

It is an important learning, how different the internal lives of people with different CFs are.[17]

3 How can we increase or decrease the strength of a feeling?

It will seem counter-intuitive but ask yourself whether it is possible to increase or diminish the strength of one of your own feelings. We may have been encouraged when young and were frightened, say, of a bully or ghost stories, not to be frightened. Did this work? Or maybe we were told to: 'Cheer up, so-and-so will pass'. Or, maybe to be respectful of granny or grandad when we simply didn't feel that way. People often say: 'I don't know, I just feel that way', as if that was the end of the story.

On other occasions, we may have been told to go for a walk/run, talk to a certain person or 'sleep on it', that is, carry out certain behaviours which would/might be incompatible with the unpleasant feelings we are undergoing. We all have evidence that changing feelings (especially negative ones) can be difficult, but is still possible. Long-term psychotherapy might have this as a goal.

NLP co-creator, Richard Bandler has proposed a simple method of changing an emotion or feeling which he called **spinning a feeling**.[18]

To learn how to increase *or* decrease the strength of a feeling, without taking drink or drugs, going for a run, having long-term therapy, or watching a movie – all of which can be time consuming, awkward or unhealthy – Richard Bandler recommended spinning a feeling. The process is simple and does require some application. It is useful in order to summon up the appropriate feeling for emotion testing.

1 Select one of the useful/desired feelings from: joy, sympathy, respect/awe, fear or objectivity/impartiality, or assertion/determination by remembering a time when you felt that feeling.

2 As you remember the times when you have felt this emotion, notice the bodily sensation that arise, especially in the chest/abdominal area.

3 Notice where the feeling starts in the body and where it goes to.

4 Spin these sensations **up your back** then **down your front**. Notice whether the feeling grows or diminishes.

5 Then enter the same feeling and spin it in the opposite direction, **up your front** and **down your back**. Notice whether the feeling grows or diminishes.

6 Use the 'increase direction' to increase any feeling you want to strengthen, and vice versa.

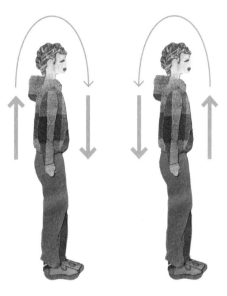

Spinning a feeling

Find out which direction increases the strength of a feeling, and which diminishes it

7 Apply this process to achieve easier access to any desirable feeling when emotion testing.

Learn to access desired and appropriate feelings. You may need to practise to become efficient, but it is useful both in the testing context, but also in life. For example, if your emotions are saying: 'I just *feel* like that, I can't help it', but your mind is saying: 'It would be good to feel differently about this issue', know that you *do* have a choice. Spin the desired feeling one way to increase it, the other way to diminish it. This will take some practise.

4 How can we recognise emotions on the face?

Chinese medicine proposes that there is one emotion associated with each Element. This is useful simplification, but in practice, for example, we often have two ends of a spectrum, both joy *and* sadness for Fire. We also have degrees of an emotion. For example, we can be extremely angry, mildly angry or just a bit angry which will all show and may be described differently. At the extremes of an emotion, people observing are likely to agree. With degrees of an emotion, observers may begin to disagree.

We also have **partial expressions** and **leaks**. Partials are where only one aspect of an emotion shows; leaks are so brief we might not see them, although video at 25 frames per second reveals them. The following tables are an attempt to encourage practitioners to observe more precisely. Our ordinary life requires that we observe accurately, but a Five Element acupuncturist is required to have even more precision. Leaks are described in more detail on page 56.

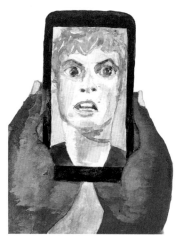

The following tables illustrate two things. The **first** describes the emotions on the **three levels of the face**, for example how do joy, anger and so on appear in the:
- **upper level** (eye brows to lower eyelids)
- **middle level** (lower eyelids to bottom of nose), and
- **lower level** (basically the mouth)?

The **second set** of tables show all of the relevant features on the **whole face, one emotion at a time**. I think both sets are useful when emotion testing and making simple observations of the chronic emotions etched onto the face.

The most useful way to read the levels of the face tables is to 'take on' each feature of the expression as you read it. It will slow you down, but you are more likely to understand and remember.

Emotions on the three levels of the face

Physical sign	Emotion
Upper level	
Eyes hard	Anger
Lower eyelids tight	Anger
Eyebrows together	Anger
Eyes soft	Sympathy/understanding/support
Head tilt	Sympathy/understanding/support
Eyes sparkling	Joy
Crows' feet	Joy
Inner corner of eyebrow/lid raised	Lack of joy
Eyes wide open, brow raised	Fear
Wrinkles across forehead	Fear
Middle level	
Cheek area dropping	Grief
Nasolabial folds increasing	Joy
Lower level	
Lips tight, tense, twitchy	Anger
Soft lips/Mouth maybe open	Sympathy/understanding/support
Mouth slightly open/flaccid	Grief/fear
Outer edges of mouth curled up	Joy
Lips curled down	Lack of joy

In the second set of tables, I list the facial and vocal features of someone who is experiencing key emotions/states. Use these to observe faces 'by emotion', for example, while watching TV or in a conversation with more than one person, where you are under no pressure to maintain the conversation. I think that observing the levels of the face first will bring better results. Experiment – but you be the judge.

Gradually you will be able to do this with patients where you are also having to maintain a conversation. When learning a new and complex skill, it is effective to learn sub-skills first and then proceed to the complex skill – just as babies, we learned to walk one sub-skill at a time. As you read the next tables, it is absolutely crucial to try the expressions on your face, ideally using a mirror. Involving your face will make a huge difference.

Facial and vocal features for the Five emotions

Fire

Joy	Crows' feet at side of eyes
	Eyes sparkling
	Nasolabial folds increasing
	Outer edges of mouth curled up
	Voice has a laugh
Lack of joy/ sadness	Outer edges of mouth turned down
	Area between eyebrows moves up
	Voice is flat

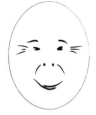

Joy

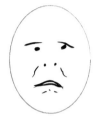

Lack of joy

Earth

Sympathy: wanting or giving	Eyes soft (can open or close slightly)
	Head tilt
	Soft lips, mouth maybe slightly open
	Voice sings
Rejecting sympathy	Verbal denial
	Bodily discomfort
	Blanking the sympathetic response

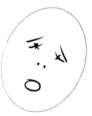

Sympathy

Metal

Grief	Cheek areas dropping
	Mouth flaccid/possibly slightly open
	General downward collapse
	Voice weeps
Receiving/ giving a positive inner quality (PIQ), see Chapter 10	Cheek areas open upwards/spread
	Eyes open slightly
	Chest area opens and moves up
	Mouth/lips firm up
Rejection of a PIQ	Explicit verbal denial
	Bodily discomfort
	Chest tightens or remains tight

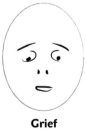

Grief

Water

Fear	Eyes open wider/brows raised
	Wrinkles in forehead
	Slight pulling backwards
	Mouth may open
	Voice groans
Lack of fear	Threat is present
	Eyes normal or fear 'leaks'
	Rest of face blank
	Voice may groan
Surprise (no fear)	Seems indistinguishable from fear on the face and the context is the differentiator; surprise is usually briefer
	Voice does not groan
Objectivity	Body/face is calm and hands may gesture from side to side, from future fantasised violation (FFV) to future fantasised safety (FFS). Objectivity is not a state to observe, but for the practitioner to express in one of the Water tests, see Chapter 11

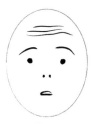

Fear

Wood

Anger	Eyes hard
	Eyebrows draw together
	Lower eyelids tight
	Lips, tight, tense, twitchy
	Voice with moments of emphasis
Appropriate assertion? – positive side of anger	Similar to above: the difference is in the 'wrongness criteria', see Chapter 12
	The intensity may be less
	Voice with moments of emphasis

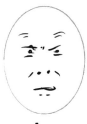

Anger

Summary of four aspects of emotions

- The **emotions are the Internal Causes of Disease.** When we experience negative emotions internally, we tend to focus mainly on our mental processes – our perceived losses, future damage, the wrong-doer, the hurt, or the lack of support – but not the concurrent and damaging bodily sensations. Treating the constitutional factor (CF) lessens the frequency and depth of these negative emotions and people often describe this in very general terms as 'feeling better in themselves'.
- **Every emotion tester also has a CF.** Knowing one's own CF and how other CFs differ can be helpful in gaining greater objectivity.
- Knowing emotions **by parts** and **by levels of the face** increases our accuracy when perceiving emotions.
- To test with ease, it is important to **develop some control over your own emotional expression**.

The next chapter covers aspects of emotion testing which are common to all emotions.

7

What is an emotion test?

The origin of emotion testing

Emotion testing is ideally a smooth process. However, like learning to walk, there are stages, stumbles, falls and gradual progress. So, the learning of emotion testing will be learning 'parts' and then putting them together. This is inevitable and hence the comparison with learning to walk.

JR Worsley demonstrated emotion testing but did not break down the stages of a test or explain how to evaluate the response to a test as normal/abnormal. What was clear was that a test involved:

- an **interaction** between practitioner and patient
- a **choice** of which Element was currently the focus
- a **test** using words and expression resonating with the Element
- **acute observation** of the patient's response, with a quick switch to
- a **judgement** as to whether the *response* was normal or abnormal – **normal** indicating that the resonating Element *was not* the CF, or **abnormal** indicating that the associated Element *was* the CF.

Although JR demonstrated, he did not explain or break down his emotion testing process. A student could learn by imitation of JR which would require many observations; or by experimenting on their own based on what they had seen JR do. I did both. I was fortunate in that, working in JR's clinic, I had access to JR's help with many of my own patients; as a clinical supervisor on JR's three-year acupuncture Licentiate courses, I had his feedback on patients in the student clinic; and doing his BAc, MAc and DrAc courses over several years, I had his CF feedback on many more patients. I considered this a privilege.

At that time, I was also a keen neuro-linguistic programming (NLP) student and was an avid 'modeller' of people's skills. **NLP modelling** is the process of recreating someone else's excellence by mastering the beliefs, the physiology and the specific thought processes or strategies that underlie the specific skill.

A small example of a behavioural model in nursing would be how to take blood from a vein (on the internet, search for: 'How to do venous blood sampling'). This is an articulate description of how to take a blood sample. Models of mental skills are similar, specifying:

- the outcome behaviour
- describing procedures
- expression
- sequence and timing
- criteria for the completion of various stages, with an appropriate level of detail.

I regarded having JR Worsley as a role model for something as new and valuable as emotion testing as a precious gift.

The stages of an emotion test and their uses

The models for testing the emotions associated with the Five different Elements are laid out in detail in Chapters 8 to 12. Most complex skills have stages, and emotion testing is no exception. Not every stage has to be enacted, because it may have already been accomplished, for example, getting rapport, but for each model to be complete, all eight possible stages need to be resolved.

The stages of emotion testing are:
1 Establish **rapport**
2 Notice or create **opportunities** to test
3 **Choose** one emotion/Element
4 **Set up to get the right content 'on the stage of the person's mind'** (pictures or words or feelings in their head/mind)
5 **Deliver the test**:
   - get the appropriate **words**, *and*
   - manifest the appropriate **expression**
6 **Observe the response**
7 **Make a judgement**
8 Note or record the **result of the test**

Each Element has a different test with different content. For some Elements, the setting up and delivery can be completed in seconds; in others it will take longer. But the pattern of testing remains the same.

The stages opposite provide a checklist. For example, at stage 5, during the delivery, finding both the right words and expression are important. Although sometimes student/practitioners can do both they are often better at one rather than the other. So, to improve their emotion testing where they are proficient at the words, you will practise the expression, or vice versa. There are multiple exercises for developing these skills in Chapters 8 to 12 on testing the Elements.

What a student can and cannot do is defined instantly in the **slow-motion emotion testing** exercise described in Chapter 13, page 106. This exercise will do three things:

1 Reveal which stages of testing a student cannot yet do
2 In real time, support learning how to perform these stages
3 Give an experience of what successful emotion testing is like

What is so useful about this exercise is that it is not just the participant in the hot seat who learns, but all participants learn. It is a gem of group learning. This is especially important for the teacher seeking to achieve results, but also for the participants.

The testing process

Once you are in rapport with the patient, there is no rule about what to do next or which Element to test first. Where to start evolves out of the conversation and rapport you have already developed. For example, if the patient immediately presents a symptom, you may find that an Earth test (giving sympathy, see Chapter 9, page 69) has been set up for you. If the patient explains that they want preventative treatment, they may have opened the possibility of a Metal test by delivering a **positive inner quality** (see testing using a PIQ, Chapter 10, page 77). If you notice the patient looking nervous and expecting you to lead, you may choose to find their biggest concern which might easily lead to a Water test. Starting with their reason for coming to treatment usually throws up options. The issue is to recognise these naturally occurring opportunities or, if not, to create opportunities.

Why is recognising the constitutional factor (CF) so important?

Your first and main intervention will usually be to treat the CF. By treating the CF, you will in turn influence other Elements via the *shen* and *ko* cycles. For example, I remember a student bringing this to my attention. On a clinical morning, she complained to me that after one treatment on the CF her patient was much better and several symptoms, which she connected with non-CF Elements, had disappeared. The student didn't understand why these non-CF symptoms had changed. I explained how the *shen* cycle carried healthy energy from one Element (the CF) to the next; this is what the *shen* cycle is about. Whilst the separation of Internal, External and Miscellaneous Causes of Disease is important, especially when giving lifestyle advice, I think it is less relevant when treating a long-term imbalance like the constitution. This the beauty of treating the CF Element.

Labels for the emotions, and their nature

The labelling of the emotions that go with the Elements has some inconsistencies. Joy is the emotion associated with Fire, but *bu li* or sadness is also relevant. Sadness, however, is not on the chart beside joy. In view of *yin/yang* theory, sadness is as significant as joy; joy is *yang* whilst sadness is *yin*.

Likewise, anger also has two sides, **appropriate** anger and **inappropriate** anger or sometimes a **lack** of anger, but in English, appropriate and inappropriate anger are not as clearly distinguished as joy and sadness. Appropriate anger is about pushing through, the forceful energy associated with growth, like a seed pushing up through the soil. (Oddly to me, Aristotle seemed to understand this: see his quote at the beginning of Chapter 12, page 97.) Again, fear is the emotion for Water, but what is its opposite? Lack of fear? That phrase is not an emotion at all; it is a statement that the patient *should* be afraid, but isn't.

The emotion of the Earth Element is overthinking or worry; what is the corresponding opposite? If we use JR's Earth emotion, sympathy, what then is its opposite: neutrality, hostility, selfishness/lack of sympathy? Grief is the emotion associated with Metal. If grief is *yin*, what is the *yang* emotion? I will explain these seeming inconsistencies Element by Element, in Chapters 8 to 12.

Testing evolves and can be endlessly refined

How long does it take to learn to emotion test? Students often do well in the CICM clinic, and by the end of the course they have the basics. But refining their skills goes on over the years. I recently met two new neighbours when walking down our road. We introduced ourselves and chatted for over five minutes. I thought she was a Metal CF and he was a Fire CF. In her case it was the facial colour, white, and something about her emotional expression and a 'holding back'. I thought he was either a Fire or Wood CF because of his immediate and strong expression of joyfulness, but given the circumstances I wasn't clear that the joy dropped so that is why I wondered about the Wood Element as well.

Those quick opinions were the result of years of experience. If I were treating them, however, I would be more thorough. My point is that increased experience speeds up an individual practitioner's testing/observation process, but simple testing and developing it remains important. In what follows, I am talking about the basic process, not how experienced practitioners develop their skills.

Evoking specific content on the 'stage of a patient's mind'

Setting up a test is making sure that everything essential is on the stage of the patient's mind ready for the delivery. By the **stage of the patient's mind** I am referring to what the patient is internally aware of at that specific moment. For example, if I asked you about your last holiday, you would have to return to the holiday to some degree to answer me and in so doing you would put aspects of the holiday on the stage of your mind, however briefly.

We do this frequently without thinking about the process. Practitioners need to get proficient at deliberately evoking specific content on the stage of the patient's mind.

Indeed, knowing how to put pleasant/useful content on the stage of our own minds is a skill to master, for no good reason other than creating a happier life. Ask yourself how well you are doing rather than asking how badly you are doing. Whatever your early experience, you can choose how to judge yourself.

Expression, delivery, observation and judgement

I use certain words, the meanings of which I hope are obvious. **Emotional expression** on the part of the practitioner accompanies the **setting up** and **delivery**. Setting up is putting whatever is necessary on the stage of the patient's mind. Delivery is the **expressive request** by the practitioner for either an **expression** of emotion or a **taking in** of an emotion. Recognising each of these involves both the right words and an expression of emotion. The practitioner's expression begins with the setting up and comes to a peak with the delivery. What follows is observation of the patient's response and the judgement as to its appropriateness.

In each of the Element chapters there are exercises for developing your emotion testing skills. I have given many options and I believe that developing your skills goes on for many years, during which it requires some deliberate effort. Practitioners start with the basics and can get better and better. JR Worsley is an obvious model.

The most similar learning situation is learning to walk in that there are several big skills and many sub-skills which need to be mastered before the overall skill of walking is accomplished. We learn to walk mainly by imitation, not instruction. So, teachers need to demonstrate repeatedly and also use the slow-motion emotion testing exercise referred to above and described in Chapter 13, page 106. Only when we have learned to walk, can we then learn to tango. There is always some way to go.

Chronic facial expressions

Chronic expressions are the residue of habitual emotions which get etched into the face from frequent repetitions, for example, the vertical lines between the eyebrows or the laugh lines at the outside of the eye and those formed in the nasolabial folds running from the lower part of the nose to the side of the mouth. These are not sufficient to spot a CF emotion, but they are indicative. In the chapters on each Element, I discuss the way each emotion shows on the face; this awareness helps enormously to interpret the 'chronics' left on the face from repetitive or held expressions.

Leaks: brief expressions of emotion on the face [19]

Another big reason for noticing 'parts' of an expression is that people tend to **leak** parts of an emotion, and for incredibly short periods. For example, some Water CFs may express fear frequently but in short bursts, as in less than a second. At that moment, fear may be appropriate, but this person does not openly express fear, which is just one of the ways of being a Water CF. Hence the word leak.

I discovered leaks while watching video of patients, one frame at a time. What I saw was, in what seemed an incredibly short time (less than a second), a flash of emotion.[20] A particular example is Water CFs who are **lack of fear**, that is people who do not usually overtly express fear, and who are often particularly competent people. These observations led me to question whether, if we were more vigilant, we could begin to see these leaks as they occur, in real time. That was when I explored **slow-motion emotion testing** as a technique, for which see Chapter 13, page 106.

How often should we test?

If a test is well formulated and the response is clear cut, maybe we only need to test once per Element. But that is a big 'if'. There is virtue, especially when a little unsure, to repeat tests, but in different contexts, especially when learning. For example, joy can occur simply upon contact, then in the context of family, a relationship or leisure. As most tests can be carried out relatively quickly, why not? Effectively then, multiple tests could well be spread throughout the initial consultation. Having a simple notation can make recording easy. For example, for a Fire test which suggests the patient is *not* a Fire CF, write: 'Fire/No' and maybe add a few words with respect to the content. If the test suggests the patient is a Fire CF, write 'Fire CF' or, when you are wavering, 'Fire CF possible'. Our capacity to test, like many practical skills, matures with use.

And, finally...

Observation of emotions has always been important in Chinese medicine. However, emotion 'testing' is different and I would question whether this existed prior to JR Worsley. It is a powerful addition to Chinese medicine.

Also, I am not qualified to say whether my description/model of what I saw JR do is what he would say he did. I suspect he wouldn't, but based on my creating a model of what I saw him do, CICM's graduates have treated many patients constitutionally with good results. As I said in a previous chapter, JR was an amazing demonstrator so to teach what I saw it was necessary to develop a model. This in no way diminishes his enormous and remarkable contribution.

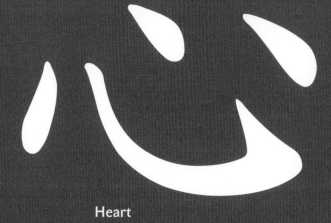

Heart

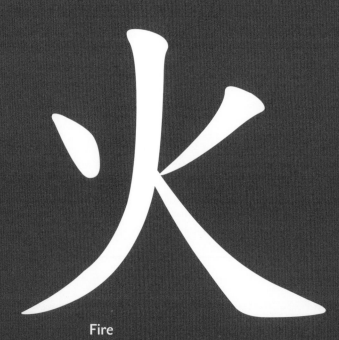

Fire

8

Testing Fire

'Sometimes your joy is the source of your smile,
but sometimes your smile can be the source of
your joy.'

Thich Nhat Hanh

'Some of you say, "Joy is greater than sorrow",
and others say, "Nay, sorrow is the greater".
But I say unto you, they are inseparable.
Together they come, and when one sits alone
with you at your board, remember that the other
is asleep upon your bed.'

Kahlil Gibran, *The Prophet*

The emotions for Fire

Testing Fire is about whether someone is a Fire CF, and not which of the
pairs of Organs – Heart and Small Intestine or Pericardium and Triple
Burner – is the more important. Treatment of someone with a Fire CF
begins on Triple Burner and Pericardium. An excellent pulse change
(everything but Pericardium and Triple Burner pulses improve) suggests
that the practitioner should continue treating those channels. If there is
little or no change, this suggests that treatment moves to Small Intestine
and Heart, which is then tested in a similar way.

Testing Fire is about *emotional* warmth and *emotional* coldness rather
than physical heat and cold. Although physical and emotional
temperature may overlap, treatment using the CF in Five Element
acupuncture is definitely about our emotions and therefore
determined by emotion testing.

In the case of Fire, whilst joy is said to be the resonating emotion, sadness (or what has been called lack of joy) is also acknowledged and it is a significant part of testing. As we will see later, it is useful to acknowledge two different emotions for each Element.

Shen is the spirit associated with Fire. If Fire is compromised, the *shen*, or the 'head of state' is compromised. One description of a disharmony of *shen* is that it manifests as anxiety, muddled thinking, and forgetfulness – the head of state is 'in a dither', not functioning well. When the *shen* is present, a person's mind is clear and settled, and the eyes are shiny and alert. Treating the Fire Element can lead to an improvement in the *shen* or mind/spirit and the patient is calmer, clearer and more composed. The emotion test for Fire is based on the state of the joy and indirectly, the *shen*.

When testing the Fire Element, the stages can often be merged in a short interaction. As long as there is rapport, the practitioner can immediately invite joy and observe the response. So, testing Fire is often brief.

The setting up criteria

The setting up criteria for each Element are reminders of what needs to be there before a test can be carried out. They are designed to assist a practitioner when starting from scratch to create the right conditions – that is, the right contents on the **stage of the patient's mind** – at the moment when the test is delivered.

The setting up criteria when testing Fire are that the practitioner:
- gives **congruent personal warmth**, or
- elicits a recent **joyous activity** on the part of the patient, then
- observes the arousal of joy followed specifically by the **natural lessening of joy**, and
- assesses both the **smooth flow** of the joy and whether there is a drop into **lack of joy/sadness**.

Congruent personal warmth involves the practitioner's capacity to express joy when encountering another person – just like when old friends meet and the joy flows smoothly and effortlessly. In the case of Fire, the emotional warmth is part of the delivery and effectively the test. Does the patient's joy rise to an appropriate level; or, does it rise up but then escalate and turn into excessive, inappropriate joy; or, does it hardly get off the ground before a lack of joy, or sadness shows through?

A drop into sadness has significance. For example, a Wood CF can express a hearty joy, but does not, in the aftermath, drop into a sadness. Instead, there is a return to their norm which indicates that their joy is not a joy arising from a Fire imbalance, but joy expressed by a Wood CF. When testing Fire, watch for the upward flow into excess or the downward drop into sadness.

The second Fire test involves a **joyous activity**. We take part in some activities simply for the pleasure of it. We meet friends just to chat, go for a picnic with the family, play with our children, play a board game, go for a walk, smell the flowers in a garden – maybe even smoke a cigarette or have a glass of wine. What are your joyous activities?

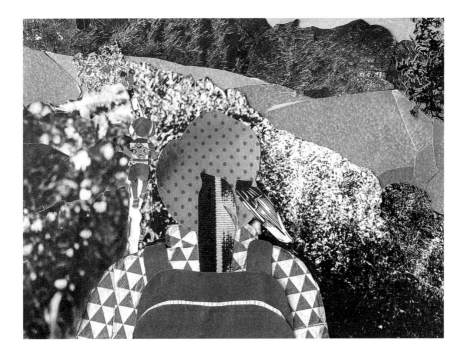

The **natural lessening of joy** is how joy rises naturally to an appropriate peak and then gradually diminishes.

Testing joy

As suggested above, there are two ways of testing Fire. The **first** is to express congruent personal warmth. For example, by saying to the patient on meeting: 'It's really good to see you' and accompanying the words with genuine joyfulness. This is an invitation for the patient also to respond with joy.

The **second** way is by asking the patient to remember a time of joyfulness, for example, a happy time with family, playing well at their favourite sport, seeing their child perform well, or getting the promotion they have been hoping for. The practitioner both expresses joy, and places a joyful memory on the stage of the patient's mind.

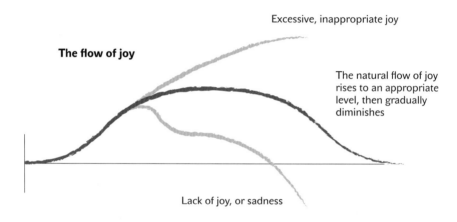

The flow of joy

Excessive, inappropriate joy

The natural flow of joy rises to an appropriate level, then gradually diminishes

Lack of joy, or sadness

Observation is the phase where the practitioner no longer expresses joy, but observes the patient's entry into joy, how it increases and how it recedes. The diagram above shows natural flow of joy. Your task is to observe whether the degree of joy is:

- **appropriate/normal** (where the joy rises and lessens smoothly)
- **sluggish/diminished** (where the joy seems unwilling to rise), or
- rises up, continues to rise and **becomes excessive**.

Accurate observation precedes a judgement, and the ability to make accurate judgements takes time to develop.

So, we have two ways of eliciting joy. Then we carefully observe the flow of joy to determine which of the three options occurred. At first, with no experience of testing, you will not know how to make this judgement. After many tests, what is normal and what is abnormal

It's really good to see you

I feel better in myself

will begin to emerge. At first, it is absolutely necessary to test without the experience of how to judge, but the more often you do the test, the more the idea of the natural lessening of joy will emerge. Then you will be able to discriminate normal joy from diminished joy from excessive joy, the latter two being indicators of a Fire CF.

You may never have thought of joy as normal or diminished or excessive. This judgement needs to be refined. Start now. Assessment of joy requires taking a keen interest in how it flows. You elicit it; you observe it; and you judge it. In so doing, you have tested the energy of the Fire Element.

Why does treatment on the Fire Element help a Fire CF?

The negative states resonating with Fire are either an ungrounded excess type of joy (as shown in the diagram opposite) where energy releases upwards leaving the person less grounded; or a downward feeling where the energy of the upper body drops, the body slumps – which we label **lack of joy** or **sadness**. Both of these are literally energy out of balance. The Fire CF, depending on the degree of imbalance, is prone to spending more time in either or both of these states and these states lead to illness.

Treatment on the Fire Element reduces the time spent in such states and thereby leads to a patient with a Fire CF saying: 'I feel better in myself' and this diminishes the occurrence of illness.

Recognising joy and sadness on the face

How do we notice a drop from joy into sadness? First, recognise joy. With **joy** what appears are:
- crow's feet wrinkles at the outside corner of the eye
- deepening of the nasolabial folds (laugh lines), and
- the corners of the mouth turn up.

This upturn of the mouth is relative. I have noticed, often in a photo, that a face expressing joy does not always have the corners of the mouth higher than the middle; they may turn up from where they started, but there is no doubt, because of the deepening of the laugh lines, that the person is expressing joy.

With **sadness** what happens is:
- the signs of joy listed above recede
- the head may drop down, and
- there is a rise in the area between the eyebrows and eyelids – try this on your own face and notice the feeling.

When joy diminishes, the **rise in the area between the eyebrows and eyelids** is a crucial observation to support the fact that the patient has dropped into lack of joy. It is easy to miss. Significantly, a person with a CF other than a Fire CF will move in and out of joy, but not drop into sadness.

Examples of recognising joy and sadness on the face

I remember JR Worsley demonstrating a very clear example. He was seeing one of my patients. Her name was Sally and she was a lively 75-year-old who had painful hands. He called her 'darling' and talked to her about going out dancing (not really a likely option for her) and she brightened up, laughed (even giggled) and her joy rocketed. As soon as this happened, he withdrew his joy and her joy plummeted into sadness, with the area between the eyebrows and eyelids shifting up. He repeated the performance twice more and she responded similarly. What he did was, I am sure, unnecessary for him, but I think it was motivated by what I would call his teacher kindness. For me, the repetition was a stunning lesson. You may wonder if this was somehow heartless, but she remembered JR positively at every subsequent visit and her hands gradually improved with treatment on the Fire Element. Also, and maybe more importantly, her joy smoothed and became less erratic.

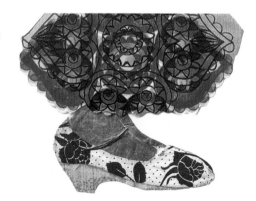

Another example was a male 35-year-old patient of mine, Andrew. It seemed like everything was a joke to him. He would look at me, with a hint of a grin on his face and then burst into a jerky, excessive joy apropos of nothing. Even asking about something neutral brought on this erratic laugh and then, as he dropped into sadness, there was a raising of the area between eyebrow and eyelids – slight, but observable.

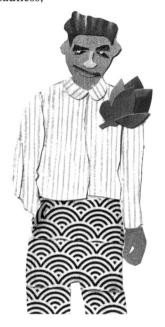

Some Fire CF patients will respond minimally to the invitation to express joy. They seem to be saying: 'No, not right now'. I had a patient who, if I teased him or joked about his condition at work or whatever, would raise a weak smile. It was as if his Heart was so heavy and his joy was so weak that 'raising joy' was very difficult. There was a noticeable change after two treatments. He came in, told me that he had a bud growing in his chest and it was turning into a flower – with a big smile on his face. He was one of my first patients and I was so naïve I had to ask him what he meant.

Fire self-training tasks

Each Element requires slightly different skills so, after the description of the tests, let's look at how you might develop the relevant testing skills. They include many things you already know how to do, but you need to define for yourself what needs to be developed.

1 **It is useful to make a list of common situations when people ordinarily experience joy**. You will be stimulating people to enter into joy so that you can observe its flow. So, part of your tool bag is knowing when, where and how easily people move into feeling joy. For example, eating a particularly delicious treat, meeting old friends, watching their children flourish, hearing positive news, your favourite team winning an important game, receiving flowers, hearing good jokes, receiving a love letter or gift, hearing praise publicly, receiving a favour, or finding something you have lost. Make a list of such times and share it with your colleagues.

2 **Make a list of appropriate compliments**, such as: 'You are looking well', 'I love the colours you are wearing' (if you do) or whatever would please the individual. You need to be sincere. Again, share your lists with colleagues and enjoy that process.

3 **Excessive and diminished joy are strong indicators**. As you notice these, the puzzle about what is appropriate or not begins to recede and you will become more comfortable making such a judgement.

4 **Bring a laugh (Five Element technical term) into your own voice**. If that is not you, listen to a person who is a Fire CF or try anything you can to find the sound. Ask a friend who is a Fire CF to help you to discover it and definitely work with someone else and get their feedback. Buy a joke book and read through it.[21] Tell the jokes as if you were expecting others to laugh and notice how your voice changes when you are finding something funny.

5 **Make a list of joyful words**, such as: fun, happy, enjoy, wow, exciting, thrilling, enthusing, electrifying – words you might use when describing an enjoyable and fun time.

6 **Practise using words or phrases from point 5, above, with 'laughter'/ joy in your voice**. It may help to say the right words like: 'Wow, that is delightful/exciting, etc', but listen to yourself and others. Possibly record your voice. Share feedback with someone else. This can be anyone who will 'play'. You might also watch comedy on TV.

7 **Practise feeling joy and sadness in yourself**. Often you need to lead with an expression of joy. How flexible are you? Can you enter joy in order to lead? Most of us do not believe we have much control over our feelings and you will find suggestions in Chapter 6, in the section on page 44 called 'How can we increase or decrease the strength of a feeling?' that can increase your control. It sounds odd, but I strongly suggest that you take this possibility seriously.

8 **Be alert for the descent from joy into sadness**. Learn to differentiate the drop out of joy into a neutral state from the drop out of joy into sadness. Joy recedes into either one or the other. This distinction is crucial and the observation needs to be sharp. Descent into a neutral state (neither joy or sadness) is usually slower than descent into sadness. The descent into sadness is often a 'drop' and is indicative of a Fire CF; the descent into neutral is not. This has to do with the vulnerability of Fire CFs. Watch for this in ordinary life.

9 Pick an exercise where you sense you have a **weakness or deficiency**. That has always been a principle of mine: not to improve your strengths, but to strengthen what you know are weaknesses or skill gaps.

Summary for Fire

- Find and accumulate situations when people **ordinarily express joy**.

- When setting up, use either **warm compliments** or **activities naturally involving joy**.

- Learn how to **spontaneously express joy yourself**, on your face and voice.

- Joyfully either give **warm compliments** or **evoke joyful memories**.

- Carefully **observe responses**, noticing the smooth (or not) flow of joy and whether the joy drops into sadness, which can be observed in the upward movement on the area on the face between the eyebrows.

- Learn to pay attention to the sensations accompanying both **your joy** and **your sadness**.

- Fire can be judged **out of balance** by a diminished expression of joy, an erratic flow of joy or a drop into sadness.

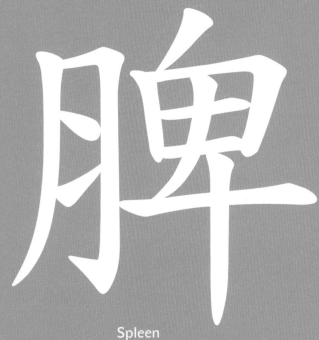

Spleen

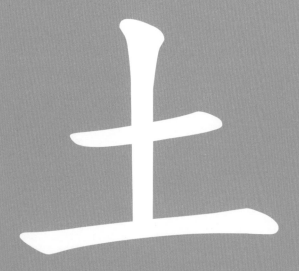

Earth

9

Testing Earth

'Love and compassion are necessities, not luxuries.
Without them, humanity cannot survive.'
Dalai Lama XIV, *The Art of Happiness*

'To be kind is more important than being right.'
The Buddha

The emotions for Earth

Unlike the Fire test, where the patient is encouraged to express
something, the Earth test asks the patient to receive/take in an
expression of **sympathy/understanding/support**. The practitioner
gives the sympathy or understanding or support and then observes
if the patient:
• takes it in (balanced and appropriate)
• resists/rejects it (not balanced or appropriate), or
• gulps it down and wants more (not balanced or appropriate).

A word first about the term sympathy/understanding/support. JR Worsley
introduced the term **sympathy** as the emotion for Earth. The translation
of the emotion associated with Earth is usually **worry**, **rumination**, or
overthinking and this is undoubtedly something Earth CFs do. Worry
and overthinking are often difficult to observe. Hence, when testing
(not described in the Classics), it is sympathy which attracts a response
and makes it more observable. I don't remember this being questioned
when I was learning and it made good sense to me. It was what Earth CFs
'wanted' (or sometimes rejected) and what the practitioner gives as a test.
This is one of JR Worsley's innovations.

When teaching, I use the term sympathy/understanding/support as it
covers all age ranges – simply because what is appropriate sympathy
varies enormously according to age. What is sympathy/understanding/

support for a five-year-old who has scraped their knee and is crying will take a very different form from a 45-year-old suffering from painful periods and again, from a 75-year-old whose knees are painful and who can't walk as far as before. All of these occurrences warrant sympathy, but the actual expression of sympathy needs to vary according to the patient's age.

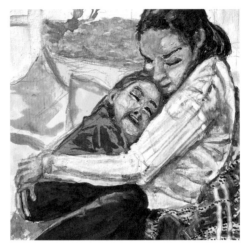

The child may need to take refuge on their parent's lap for a few moments and maybe even have their knee 'kissed better'. Someone suffering from painful periods needs help from a practitioner who clearly understands pain, and an older person needs a practitioner who knows something about pain *and* what it is like thinking it will never go away. Hereafter, I will just use the one word, sympathy.

The setting up criteria

One could think that eliciting a complaint is easy. After all, patients come for acupuncture because they have a problem or complaint. It should be easy and, in a way it is, but you still need to be careful about what you understand the complaint to be. That is why in the setting up criteria we refer to the wound and the inner wound.

The setting up criteria for sympathy are:
- there is a **wound** (often the same as the complaint)
- there is an **inner wound** (the consequence of the initial wound/complaint)
- the wound/complaint is **recent** or **ongoing**
- it **can't easily be changed**.

Clarifying the wound and inner wound

One of the first steps is to attempt to be sure what the wound and/or inner wound is. The wound is what the person complains about, for example: 'My foot hurts', 'I have migraines', 'Someone left their car blocking my driveway'. You get the inner wound by understanding (or eliciting) what that means for the person.

For example, a late train may mean nothing or it might have serious implications. For example: 'I missed my connection and as a consequence missed the lecture'. So, what? 'Well, there was a question on the exam specifically about the subject of that lecture and I failed the exam as a result.' It is not always easy to evaluate the validity of a complaint. Getting the inner wound, which is the negative effect on the patient, is not crucial except that it helps the practitioner evaluate a complaint.

Testing sympathy

The test is to give appropriate sympathy. **Appropriate** means specifically taking age into consideration, which will vary the nature of the sympathy given. The practitioner also needs to take into consideration whether the patient has what appears to be the stated complaint (wound) or the inner wound. The question is then: 'Does the person take the sympathy in?'. **Taking in** means accepting the sympathy, appreciating it and being satisfied with it. **Not taking in** the sympathy usually manifests by verbally rejecting it (less common) or (more common) complaining more and more as if the initial sympathy was a signal to want more and more. It is a subtle judgement which requires giving sympathy on many occasions and noticing the differing responses.

Examples exploring sympathy

I remember an older lady, Jenny, whose presenting complaint was pain in her wrist; she called it arthritis. For clarity, I asked her what she couldn't do as the result of the pain. She looked confused. I asked if she could lift a heavy teapot. She looked uncomfortable and said: 'Yes'. I was becoming aware that she wanted help, but it wasn't just for the wrist. Not uncommonly, she didn't know how to present her complaint which was more about becoming isolated and not feeling she could ring up friends and family. She said, in the end, that there was nothing she could do for anyone anymore. She was a 'helper' and getting older she had lost her ability to get out and do the helping work she had done before.

Earth CFs are often **helpers** and losing this capacity can be distressing. She wasn't sufficiently aware or articulate enough to make that her complaint and a doctor may not have taken that complaint seriously and may not have prescribed drugs. So, that was not formally a test, but arose from trying to clarify the complaint and knowing how out-of-balance sympathy plays out in practice.

Another older female, referred by her son, was unsure of her complaint. On the surface, it was tiredness. In the end, it came down to not being appreciated by her husband and three sons. They took her for granted, leaving their clothes on the floor for her to pick up, expecting meals and washing up to be done, with no acknowledgement or thanks. She had done something that Earth CFs often do. They help others to such a degree that they get taken for granted and then never receive the appreciation they once received or hoped for.

The above examples illustrate why there is both the wound and the inner wound. Practitioners need to take the surface wound as important, but realise there is possibly another deeper wound, which, if known, makes treatment make more sense. In the case of the lady who was referred by her son, treatment helped her understand the issue and the goal of treatment then moved from alleviating the arthritis in her hands, which was happening anyway, to letting her husband and sons know that she was not their servant and they needed to pick up their own underwear.

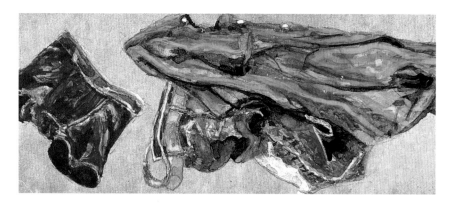

Rarely, Earth CFs are not helpers, but instead **reject sympathy**. A friend referred a male patient to me. The patient was well off, in his early 40s and had moved out of his home, leaving his wife with two teenage boys. He would return to his home once or twice a week, but otherwise he worked in the day and what he called 'cruised' in the evenings in Soho. Cruising meant picking up prostitutes, having sex, sometimes twice in one evening. He was explicit about his sexual behaviour, but it was not his complaint and definitely not up for discussion. Many of his presenting complaints, aches and pains, improved and I consistently treated him at the spirit level. I heard later from my friend who had referred him that he was again living at home. Occasionally, Earth CFs reject sympathy.

Another Earth CF who rejected sympathy was an older man, Gerald, who, at end of treatment took 20 minutes plus to get dressed and tie his shoelaces. He refused help and we were in a two-bed clinic so his remaining in the treatment room severely disrupted the flow of patients. After several treatments, I explained and asked if he could help *me* by allowing me to help him. Under those conditions, he obliged.

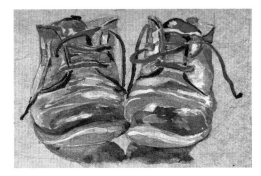

Earth self-training tasks

1 **Work first on your voice: both the tone of voice and the words people use when they are feeling sympathy, understanding or support**. Think of real statements you can make where you genuinely feel sympathy and do so. Think of people/organisations in the world for whom you feel supportive. Take phrases like: 'I am so sorry to hear that' or: 'I do understand how difficult that is'. Let your voice sing, allowing it to roll up and down as if singing a lullaby. Make a scale from 1 to 5 where 1 is 'a bit of a sing' and 5 is 'a whole lot of sing'. Do a 1, then a 2, then a 3, then a 4 and finally a 5. Do this a sufficient number of times that you will have developed 'expressive flexibility' with this particular sound. If you can do it with a friend/colleague, even on the phone, do so. Make it fun. Review this regularly until you can make your voice sing with ease.

2 **Learn to look/be sympathetic and understanding**, so others look at you and instantly know you are feeling that way. Use a mirror and involve your face and body: tilt your head, open your mouth slightly, move closer and spread your hands or reach out to touch.
If necessary, use a model, someone you know who is expressive in this way. To help, as you do this, imagine someone who you genuinely feel sympathy for. Use others for feedback. If you are an Earth CF, this might not be necessary.

3 The better that you can remember where you were when you naturally felt **sympathy/understanding/support**, the better you will know it in your body and the better you will recognise it in others.

4 **Make a list of at least 15 areas/incidents where sympathy/ understanding/support would be appropriate**: people who have less advantages than you, such as refugees; children born with obvious health disadvantages; life situations where your patients may be suffering prejudice, hardship, personal crises; people working as carers in stressful situations, or (similar to Wood) where someone has been treated unfairly or without thought. This may be by neighbours, friends, organisations, Network Rail, the local council, a particular political party, the college you are attending, other drivers, your boss, other people's pets, members of the same organisation, and so on. You may need to ask others doing the same exercise to get a full list.

5 **Get a study buddy** for the exercises or for demonstrating your expression. Swap experiences. Ideally, work together with others on the above exercises; their feedback will help you and vice versa.

6 **Pick an exercise** where you sense you have a **weakness or deficiency**. That has always been a principle of mine: not to improve your strengths, but to improve what you know are weaknesses or skill gaps.

7 I hesitate to recommend Google, but in the case of sympathy, if you search for 'expressions of sympathy' you will find an impressive number of suggestions. Your judgement will be tested; it can help you develop a sense of appropriateness.

Summary for Earth

- **Sympathy/understanding/support** is used instead of overthinking, or worry.

- When setting up, the practitioner searches for a complaint, looks for the **wound**, the **inner wound** and ascertains that it is **recent** or **ongoing**.

- It helps understanding, but it not absolutely necessary to get clarity about what is the wound and inner wound.

- Sympathy/understanding/support must be **delivered congruently**: voice singing, facial expression (head tilt, mouth soft or slightly open, maybe a touch).

- If when manifesting sympathy, you find you get stuck in it, develop a pattern of any sort to **clear the feeling** – see example below.

- The response can be judged:
  - **normal** (congruent acceptance of the sympathy)
  - **rejection of the sympathy** (an indication of Earth weakness), or
  - **acceptance and immediate, extended complaining** soliciting more sympathy/understanding/support.

- Work on your voice, sympathetic appearance, appropriate time for sympathy, and work on expression with others for feedback.

Clearing a feeling Feeling sympathy can easily cross over into 'picking up' another's symptoms. If you find you feel worse after a day's practice or you know specifically you have picked up a patient's symptom do the following. Stand and raise up on your toes and then drop with a thud onto your heels. Start with ten drops and check how you feel. Continue until you are free of the feeling.

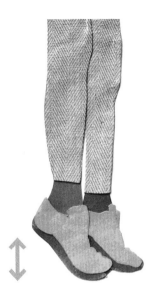

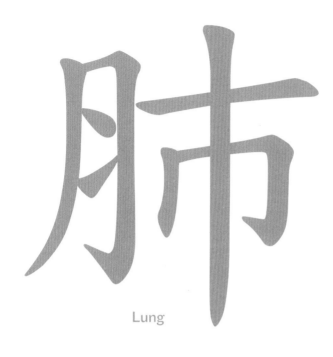

Lung

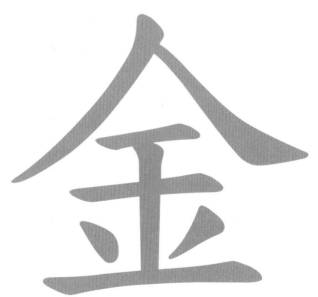

Metal

10

Testing Metal

'How lucky I am to have something that makes saying goodbye so hard.'
Winnie the Pooh

'Grief: It batters the immune system, leaving you depleted and vulnerable to infection. The heartbreak of grief can increase blood pressure and the risk of blood clots. Intense grief can alter the heart muscle so much that it causes "broken heart syndrome", a form of heart disease with the same symptoms as a heart attack.'
webmd.com

The emotions for Metal

With Fire, sadness is the *yin* emotion alongside joy. Metal seems only to have one emotion: grief. However, Metal has a positive emotion as well, for which we don't have a single and appropriate label. To me this is an unfortunate omission, which has confused the testing process. So, before describing the tests, we need to clarify the two emotions.

With Metal, the emotion is grief, where the emphasis is on what is missing after a loss. The alternative emotion is how we feel when dealing with life's losses or difficulties and respond positively. English does not have a single word for this emotion, but some possibilities are: strength, grit, tenacity, resoluteness, or gutsiness.[22] Any of these are candidates as they all suggest a positive response to real or potential loss and seeing a difficult situation through. Feeling grief with a loss is appropriate.

We can generalise and label this as a **positive inner quality** or **PIQ**. So, Nelson Mandela's positive response on emerging from prison was not grieving for how much of his life he lost. Instead he was positive. What was the right word for that positivity after such a long loss of freedom? Practitioners need to find a 'right' word or phrase for an individual patient's positive response to loss. This is a PIQ: deliver it. Usually, once we have that label, the delivery with respect is straightforward.

We will start with the grief test and come back to the more positive test.

Recognising grief

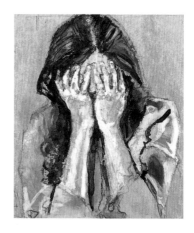

In a patient's history, there will many instances of losses on all levels: physical, mental and spiritual. There can be losses of possessions, money or goods of all sorts. There can be physical, emotional or mental losses, for example, strength, friendships or mental capabilities. There can be losses affecting the spirit, maybe described as losses of confidence, happiness or purpose. It may be a stronger test to choose a loss which is not just physical, but also internal in some sense. Whatever touches a person more deeply, will have a stronger effect.

When testing, you test because you don't know how a patient will respond. So, it is interesting to know that the loss a Metal CF feels can turn out to be either the kind of loss that Fire, Earth, Wood and Water CFs feel, but *in addition* it is a feeling of loss which is hard to express. Paradoxically, Metal CFs can feel loss, when nothing has been lost. It is not a physical object; it is not a mental capacity; it is not a spiritual quality that is specifiable. It is an *unspecifiable* loss. Just something is missing, but what?

So, it is common that the person with a Metal CF behaves or feels as if they have lost something but is not articulate about what it is they have lost. This is a Metal CF's grief. Superficially, this is irrational, so you do not hear a Metal CF saying: 'I have lost something, but I don't know what it is', simply because that doesn't make sense. But they can still feel/ behave that way. This is the puzzle of being a Metal CF. On the face of it, illogical or even absurd.

So what, that's gone, who cares?

Me feeling loss, no way!

Testing grief

With this test, the question is whether the person can go into grief and come out of the other side. The procedure to test grief has three brief phases:

1 Remind the patient of the pleasure or satisfaction – the good feelings that were associated with the person/animal/position – before the loss.
2 Encourage them to re-enter those positive feelings by remembering or associating into how it used to be.
3 When they have re-entered the positive feelings associated with the loss (what is now gone), say something like: 'And now sadly, that (whatever is missing) is gone', or similar words, brief and emphasising the loss.

The process sounds harsh, and it is deliberately so, in order to test the ability to feel grief *and* to let go. Non-Metal CFs can go into grief and come out in a way that those who are Metal CFs find hard. So, observe the response. Can the person:

- **roll with the grief**, that is, go into it, feel it, and come out again, or do they
- **get stuck in grief** (not likely), or do they
- **brush it off** as if: 'So what, that's gone, who cares?'.

The majority of Metal CFs will be brusher-offers: 'Me feeling loss, no way!'.

In my experience, this test works to identify Metal CFs. As I said above, non-Metal CFs can roll with it, go into the feeling of grief, and come out. Metal CFs will become uncomfortable, the most common response being to bottle up and just not go there, manifesting an apparent indifference, in order not to feel uncomfortable. It can be useful for the practitioner to change the subject and lead the patient away into another subject. But the Metal CF may well have done that by themselves.

Although this test works, I tend not to use it, because, fortunately, there is a much kinder, more patient friendly alternative.

Testing using a positive inner quality (PIQ)

A preferable test is to find a time when the patient had a struggle with a loss. For example, when studying and running out of money, losing a loved one, losing a beloved pet, losing a job suddenly, losing status abruptly or losing anything that was highly valued – these are all situations of loss.

This is where the description of emotions in Chinese medical theory is lacking. Fire has joy and its opposite, sadness. Metal has grief and 'something' which is the opposite, but for which we have no explicit label. So, if you take expressions of strength or virtue whilst under the stress of loss – the opposite to or response to the feeling loss – we could add even more qualities to the list above: grit, kindness, generosity, objectivity, strength, passion, fearlessness, compassion, gratitude, determination, 'stick-to-it-ive-ness', hope, awe, optimism, benevolence, and so on. Because the PIQ does not have a specific label, the practitioner provides it.

It is important to note that the PIQ has, explicitly or implicitly, a state of loss/grief which the PIQ is in contrast with. Nelson Mandela could have expressed grief over the years of loss of freedom when emerging from prison, but instead he was positive. When suffering a loss, Metal CFs can simply 'go under' or they can react positively, as it were, against the loss. The practitioner's skill is to find that response, label it as a PIQ and deliver it to find out whether the patient can take it in. *The issue is how the Metal CF responds.* Non-Metal CFs can take it in; Metal CFs will find it hard as their Receiver of *qi* energy from the Heavens is impaired. They are consummate brusher-offers: 'Me special? No way!'.

The stages of a PIQ test

1 The practitioner elicits a **brief account of the loss** and the patient's **positive response**.

2 While listening to the account of the loss, the practitioner formulates a **short verbal description of a PIQ manifested by the patient** during the time after the loss. For example, resilience, courage, endurance, compassion, or purposefulness. These are **positive** (hence admirable), **inner** (not in any way physical) and a **quality** that can be **directly attributed to the person**. These PIQs are the counterbalance to grief, as joy is to sadness. On occasions, the PIQ may be very difficult to find,

but not usually, because Metal CFs are often conscientious and do manifest good qualities.

3 The practitioner then **attributes the PIQ to the patient**. For example: 'You showed compassion under extremely difficult circumstances' or: 'To hang in there for that length of time shows to me that you have courage and real compassion'. (Think again of Nelson Mandela, his loss when being in prison and what you could say to him upon being released from prison.) It is necessary to carry out the process without hesitation.

4 The **final stage**, after the succinct and direct attribution of the PIQ, is to observe whether the patient **takes it in** with comfort or ease or **looks awkward**, **denies the PIQ** or simply **appears not to hear it**. The difference in response between Metal CFs and non-Metal CFs is usually unmistakable. If a person takes the PIQ in smoothly, they are not a Metal CF, whereas denying, choking up or simply blanking suggests they are a Metal CF. The blocking off or stagnation in the chest area, is a visual clue. Whilst the verbal brushing-off will be clear, what is easy to miss is this tightening of the chest which is how the patient blocks the acceptance of the PIQ.[23]

Developing the degree of verbal articulation and quick thinking needed when formulating the PIQ is challenging. Initially most practitioners are not fluent at formulating PIQs, but it comes with practise.

To recap Having listened to the person's struggle, the task is to verbalise a PIQ the patient manifested and then deliver it back to them. For instance, someone who was betrayed or badly let down by a partner/friend might initially feel loss, and then respond differently by expressing compassion towards that person. Briefly reiterate the disappointment, then say: 'You showed real compassion (or courage, sensitivity, love)' – whatever you feel is appropriate. The question then is: 'Does the patient take it in?'. As described above, the response will usually be distinctive. The skill is knowing what to look for.

Most people do not have this skill naturally. Indeed, it surprises me that in many cultures, although people often express warmth (Fire), they much less frequently express what might be called respect or admiration, except for displays of physical skill or some extreme expertise. Practise is necessary to be able to deliver PIQs fluently.

Examples involving PIQs

My own experience as a Metal CF provides an example which also showed me that not all treatment requires needles: the right life experience, in the right circumstances can function as a treatment. I was once in a large NLP training with 80+ participants. I was already an acupuncture practitioner and knew I was a Metal CF, but more from being told than any genuine insight. At one moment, the whole group turned to me, and one person publicly gave me a clear PIQ in front of everyone. I was just about to deny it, pushing it away and do what I would always have done when I thought: 'This is a positive inner quality. I can take it in.'

With effort, I denied myself my habitual response which was discomfort and deflection. Instead, I did my best to take it in and did so to a much

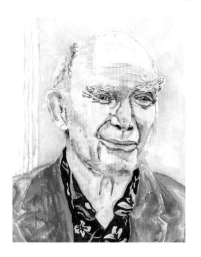

greater extent than usual. I ended up in tears pleased that I had behaved totally differently, embarrassed by my tears yet feeling obvious satisfaction at being acknowledged. I would associate what is called Receiving *qi* energy from the Heavens with the noticeable movement of *qi* in my chest area. I did manage to say: 'Thank you'. The Lung function is to Receive *qi* energy from the Heavens and that is what my Lungs did, however awkwardly. That incident functioned like a treatment. It enabled me to be more receptive to what non-Metal CFs take for granted, that is, being able to Receive PIQs from the Heavens. One practice for Metal CFs, recorded in *Healing your Emotions*, is to give PIQs to others until they become acutely aware of their own needs.[24]

A 35-year-old female patient was treated at the CICM teaching clinic. After five treatments, she was not changing. None of three supervisors, including me, thought she was a Metal CF and without much progress she had persisted with treatment for several sessions. I was her supervisor on treatment 5 and I told her how much I appreciated her commitment to treatment and her faith in us. Unintentionally, I had delivered a PIQ. She started to tear up and I realised what I had done. She had demonstrated difficulty in Receiving *qi* energy from the Heavens. She progressed rapidly with treatment on Metal.

So, what does a practitioner do when the person with a Metal CF blanks out or denies the PIQ? Move on quickly, diminish the discomfort and treat Metal. Usually, there is no need to worry about their discomfort; it will be brief and the value to the treatment is immense.

Later on, test again and look for a difference, that is, more ability to Receive *qi* energy from the Heavens which is a powerful marker that the Lungs are improving. You may well have noticed improvements in the patient's complaints, but you might discover that the ability to Receive *qi* energy from the Heavens is also a significant and powerful indicator. This is what we often refer to – in the case of Metal CFs – as 'feeling better in ourselves'. Being better able to Receive *qi* energy from the Heavens creates emotional healing.

Another Metal CF patient was modest to an extreme degree. She was intellectually more than competent and was working on a graduate degree when she came for treatment. She had a grant but was also working part-time to support a younger brother, both of them having been abandoned by a single mother. When I appreciated her for her personal effort while at the same time caring for her brother, she cut me off and denied these PIQs. Taking in a PIQ was not yet an option for her, but she showed her CF.

Metal self-training tasks

1 First, ask yourself how often you deliberately do your best and no one notices.

2 Because you want to learn to deliver a **positive inner quality (PIQ)**, it would be helpful to **write in your notebook a list of what you understand to be PIQs** and what might incline you to attribute them to someone. Think of qualities in others that you admire and respect which are not physical attributes and make a list. For example:
   – Think of the UK in 2020 in the middle of the coronavirus pandemic. Think of the hospital staff who frequently risked their lives to help others. What PIQs did they manifest?
   – We admire athletes for their physical performance, but we also admire them for commitment, skills, training hard, and teamwork which are not just physical but also mental or psychological
   – However, the majority of your patients will not be top athletes so consider the qualities of ordinary people who under stress respond positively, resourcefully and with admirable qualities. Starting with

people you know, make a list of their possible PIQs. Think of when they have been under duress and formulate the PIQs they manifested until you are fluent with PIQs. Include children in your examples.

3 **Deliver some of the PIQs in ordinary life** and notice peoples' responses. Beside it being a satisfying thing to do, the main purpose here, of course, is for testing. Share your thoughts and list them with other emotion testers. This will help you to respond fluently, which is an important learning issue. (Remember: you are thickening the myelin sheath of the relevant circuits in your brain, the basis of habit and fluency.)

4 Remember times when you have been impressed, not necessarily pleased, but **impressed by what someone did**. They may have been sensitive (to others' feelings), brave (being frightened, but standing up for their own or others' rights), kind (when it would have been easy to not bother), generous (such as committing 10% of their income to others), fair (when it would easier to be unfair), and so on. In each case:
   – **put into words** what impressed you, and
   – **imagine delivering what you noticed** (the PIQ) to the person
      in question.

5 Work on your voice to achieve a **tone of respect/admiration**. It is not a joyful or happy tone. It is one reflecting: 'I'm impressed and I noticed'. Often, this involves the upper body moving back slightly and the voice rising slightly upwards. List some respectful compliments (see point 2 above) and say them out loud.

6 Remember times where **you admired another person** – someone being generous, a skilful performance, an act of kindness or maybe selfless caring. Express it in words in a tone demonstrating admiration or respect. It could be as simple as telling the person who cooked the meal how good it was. Or telling someone at work how well they handled a tricky situation. Or how well/kindly/skilfully your child behaved. (Notice that is it easier with children than with adults to deliver PIQs.) Get the voice tone just right for respect. Do not confuse this with an expression of joy. Expressing awe or respect does not involve a smile.

7 **Practise entering a feeling of admiration or respect**. Do this as a thought experiment. Think of what you admire/respect and let the feeling rise up. Grief has a downward path and admiration/respect has upward one. The feeling can and should rise up through the chest. Having done it as a thought experiment, now do it in practice. If you

are a Metal CF, this will be more difficult, but all the more useful for you. Take a person you know well, formulate a PIQ and deliver it. Repeat until you are smooth. If you practise respecting others, it gets easier to then respect yourself so there is also an aspect of self-healing.[25] This activity is both preparation for being able to test Metal, but should also help by exercising a Metal quality (giving respect) to help your own Metal Element.

8 In daily life, whenever you chat to someone, **find ways of asking if life has been easy lately or has there been difficulties, stress or problems**. When people respond with any of these, see if you can quickly (as per the previous exercises) formulate a PIQ – something about how they behaved which was admirable. Then, where you can, deliver the PIQ. Deliver with respect and matter-of-factly, then pay careful attention to their response. Did they take it in; were they uncomfortable and hesitated, resisted or blanked what you said? With practise (and not without), you will become fluent.

9 **Pick an exercise** where you sense you have a **weakness or deficiency**. That has always been a principle of mine: not to improve your strengths, but to strengthen what you know are weaknesses or skill gaps.

Summary for Metal

- There are two ways to test Metal: one by **inviting the patient into grief**, the other by **delivering a positive inner quality (PIQ)**. The former works, but is less patient friendly; the latter is preferable.

- Most of us need to practise formulating PIQs.

- **Develop the right voice tone** for delivering the PIQ.

- Practise **entering a state of respect**.

- The patient either **obviously takes in** the PIQ or **struggles with taking it in/rejects it**.

賢

Kidney

水

Water

11

Testing Water

> 'I learned that courage was not the absence of fear, but the triumph over it. The brave man is not he who does not feel afraid, but he who conquers that fear.'
>
> Nelson Mandela

> 'Fear is the main source of superstition, and one of the main sources of cruelty. To conquer fear is the beginning of wisdom.'
>
> Bertrand Russell

The emotions for Water

Water presents a different testing challenge. Water CFs tend to develop in one of two ways. Either they:
- **feel afraid overtly and excessively** and they are unable to hide it, or
- they **live fearlessly**, at least on the surface, and rarely if ever seem to be frightened, even though internally this may not be true.

As a result, early on the practitioner needs to observe whether there is noticeable fear showing. This difference is not absolute, but important. No other Element is quite the same.

Early in my career, I more frequently missed the second type of Water CF – those who, on the surface, never seem to be frightened. Knowing how to make this distinction can make testing more effective. So, what is the difference?

When a Water CF doesn't show fear, fear is still present, but it does not exist on the surface. Indeed, the person may be quite skilled – whilst holding fear in the body – in appearing confident or fearless. It may not be clear whether they are *consciously* or deliberately behaving confidently or whether, as is often the case, when asked: 'Are you frightened?', they would say: 'No', and mean it. They are often successful in the world, especially in business where fear leads them to make careful, skilful assessment of risks. This unconscious tendency serves them well in many areas of life.

The downside of such lack of fear is **paralysis**. It is a matter of degree. For example, Water CFs who have a lack of fear may find an ideal partner, but they are never able to move in together. As one Water CF said to me: 'How do you ever know whether you can share a bathroom, eat the same meals or go to bed at the same time? I prefer things the way they are now. She has her flat, I have mine.' This fear-driven wariness, in excess, can be paralysing; in moderation, it is often a strong internal motivator.

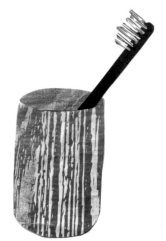

When a patient is showing fear, the diagnostic challenge is to assess whether the fear is a **Water fear**, that is, due to a weakness of the Water Element, or an ordinary fear brought about by very challenging circumstances where good sense indicates appropriate fear. This situation requires a different test; hence there are two Water tests, depending on the initial presentation.

The above distinction requires an early assessment. Is this patient clearly frightened, and showing it, or do they seem positive, confident and without fear? Making this initial assessment as soon as possible is important as it indicates which test to carry out. The two tests are not alternatives as with Metal, but using one or the other depends on how the patient presents. This means testing Water may take longer.

The setting up criteria

The setting up criteria covers both tests. They are:
- **threat** (which tells us something bad might happen)
- **future fantasised violation** or **FFV** (the 'something' that is bad)
- **future fantasised safety** or **FFS** (that the something bad does *not* happen)
- information about the likelihood of both FFV and FFS.

Recognising fear on the face

It is helpful to be clear about how fear manifests on the face:
- the eyes open wider, brows raised
- wrinkles appear across the forehead
- there is an intake/holding of breath
- the mouth may drop slightly open.

The eyes are probably the most reliable indicator.

Testing fear: set up and delivery

The **first test** is when **fear is plainly visible**. The ears are the sense Organ resonating with Water. Ears allow us to hear. The test is whether the person can 'hear' both sides of the apparent threat when presented objectively, that is, its likelihood of leading to the:
- future fantasised violation (FFV), or
- future fantasised safety (FFS).

This is best done *as if* you had a flipchart (you won't) and were presenting the options, an FFV or FFS, in a dissociated way. **Dissociated** means that the practitioner's state is neutral, and makes no assumption one way or the other.

Let us say the patient is expressing fear about an upcoming visit to the doctor to receive test results for a cancer biopsy. Your emotion test is already set up. The test is simply for the practitioner to present (or re-present) the possible outcomes as objectively as possible, that is, one after the other – preferably the FFV first and the FFS second. The possibilities are expressed neutrally, whatever the odds are, that is, no bias toward either option.

The test is *not* whether the patient is afraid, but whether the patient can listen. The ears are the sense Organ associated with Water. **Can listen** means the patient sits there and hears the options. **Can't listen** means the patient will squirm, turn away, close their eyes, put their hands up as if to protect themselves, or any behaviour suggesting: 'I don't want to listen'. The difference is usually clear. Can't listen suggests the person is a Water CF. Can listen suggests that they are not a Water CF, but are simply being appropriately fearful.

The **second test** is when the patient **shows no fear**, verbally or facially. In this case, setting up the test entails finding something that the patient should show at least some fear about, then raising the issue emphasising the potential threat and FFV. As the patient has come because of a complaint (potential threat), it is usually possible to find a sufficient threat. The practitioner expresses the fear on behalf of the patient, widening the eyes, pulling the body slightly back and holding the breath. For the patient, the fear is nowhere near the surface; it does not show on the outside and only appears extremely briefly if the practitioner scares the person. So, the fear, if it is there, will often appear as a **leak**; this makes it important when using the test to be ready for a very brief flash of fear. Alternatively, if the patient says: 'Yes, I am worried/frightened of that' and shows some fear, but demonstrates they can hear/listen, they are probably not a Water CF.

Examples showing fear and lack of fear

First, the Water CFs who are **obviously fearful**. Molly was a fearful type of Water CF. She was 45 and did office work from home. Her main complaint was: 'Fear of going out'. When asked what she was afraid of, she said her neighbourhood was dangerous. She worked from home to avoid going out. She did go out, to shop and visit family, but the journeys were unpleasant and she spent freely on taxis to avoid being on the street. Could Molly listen to reassurance of any sort?

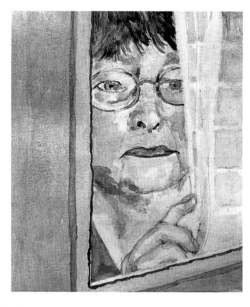

No. She just squirmed and looked away.

Jack was a similar patient. He was 39 and had no complaint. Jack was clearly nervous from the beginning. When asked why he came, he said he had nothing wrong with him, he had just been told by his wife to come (his wife was already a clinic patient), but he insisted there was nothing wrong with him. Jack already looked terrified, his eyes were held wide open, and his breathing was shallow (Water CFs often cannot breathe deeply).[26]

You must be really scared

No I'm not. You're going to help me

A **lack of fear** patient is different. A patient I had years ago presented in a wheelchair and when I entered the room, he announced that he had MS and it was the fastest growing his consultant had ever seen – six weeks and he was in a wheelchair. I said to him, pulling back and expressing fear by widening my eyes: 'You must be scared. Your condition is very, very serious and your consultant is correct.' His response was to smile and say: 'No, I'm not. You're going to help me', with no apparent expression of fear. (Looking back, I may have missed the leak.) This is what is called lack of fear: the situation is scary, but the patient seems untouched by fear. Treatment confirmed the diagnosis.

There is a tendency to avoid such a test, where you deliberately attempt to scare the patient. It may feel brutal, but remember, getting the diagnosis correct is the practitioner's responsibility. Also, eliciting fear can be over in seconds and your skill, as well as eliciting fear, is also to return the situation quickly to what might be called normal. This is generally easy. Patients who are lack of fear, under provocation will show fear but only briefly (a challenge for the practitioner to even notice) and they return quickly to their norm, that is a lack of fear.[27] You have to experience this to believe it, especially if you are a kind, thoughtful and sensitive practitioner. All I can say is that you need to be ruthless to be compassionate and the 'patient disruption' quickly returns to the patient's norm, that is, lack of fear.

Patients showing a lack of fear often do not *consciously* experience fear in the way a non-Water CF would. As a result, they can be difficult to recognise. On a CF day at CICM, where different CFs describe their inner experience, one lack of fear Water CF described this process with great clarity. He was both a practitioner and had known what his CF was for years.

Water CFs may **reframe their fear**, like one lady who once told me that she frequently drove down the M4 at over 100 miles per hour in her boyfriend's car. I questioned the good sense in doing this and she said: 'No, I love it. I really feel alive'. So, I then asked if she ever felt frightened. She immediately said: 'Oh yes, I go to scary movies and sit in the front row and I am terrified': both inappropriate lack of fear and inappropriate fear. She also bungee jumped. This phenomenon is more common than we might expect.

Another example was a lady in her 80s who was partially blind. She had scars on her wrists and hands and I asked her about them. She said: 'Oh, when I'm cooking, because I can't see so well, I often burn my hands'. I asked if there was no one who could help her in the kitchen. She said: 'Oh, my daughter wants me to move in with them and she would cook for me, but I like my independence.' If people practise not feeling fear for long enough, they become good at it and can do something frightening with their attention not on the fear, but somewhere else. There are many outwardly successful Water CFs in the world.

How does this happen? I once had a revealing conversation with a Water CF who had a lack of fear. In the course of treatment, he became more conscious of when he felt fear and speculated about its origin. He said as a young boy (and already a Water CF) his father would encourage him to do what he felt were scary activities, like playing football with older boys, jumping in the deep end of the pool and joining a wrestling class, none of which he wanted to do. He did what his father encouraged, became superficially brave, but lost contact with his deeper feelings and ended up with chest pains which Water treatment resolved. As he improved, however, he began to feel fear again and later he realised that fear was an important signal and not to be ignored.

My understanding is that if you **exclude** or even **diminish awareness of fear** from your consciousness, you begin to crave experiences that do stimulate you and that requires increasing risk. Evel Knievel, who famously rode motorbikes through the air and over many buses in a row, made a living from his CF and, curiously, broke 433 bones in the process, bones being the body part associated with Water. He had to be a Water CF.

Water self-training tasks

1 First **make lists of things that most people find scary**, for example, running out of money, being hurt in a car crash, your children's health being threatened, your dwelling being broken into, losing your job, having a fluctuating health problem, catching the covid virus, not knowing where your next meal is coming from or where you will sleep tonight. Brainstorm with others and make the list as long as you can about what, for anyone, might be scary.

2 **Learn to see fear on the face**. See fear both when frightened and when, in a diminished expression, it gets etched into the face. I am not suggesting you can't see fear, just that you can become better at it. Chronic fear is a residue of acute fear appearing habitually. The clues are, without any fear stimulus being present: the eyes opening widely with eyebrows raised, wrinkles across the forehead, an intake of breath, the mouth opening slightly and the breath being held.

3 It is helpful early on to learn to express both a **state of objectivity** and a **state of fear**, one for the first and the other for the second test:
   – The objective state is as if you had no interest other than to approach the truth. Your feelings are completely neutral, as if the choice is important, but you have no personal investment one way or the other. This may not be a familiar state, because most of the time in life we have a bias. But on this occasion, we don't and that must come across to the patient. Practise until you are proficient. Let colleagues judge you.
   – The second state to express is one of fear, as with the MS patient above. You may be familiar with the fear state. If not, think of scary things and let yourself experience fear and study it. Eyebrows go up, eyes widen, and the head may pull backwards whilst breathing pauses. If necessary, fake it until you are fluent. Practise 'degrees of'. You do this not for fun, but to become a better practitioner.

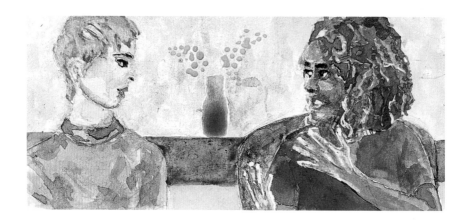

– Work on the words separately and then combine them. The words, if necessary, would be questioning, for example: 'What?' or 'Really?' or 'That's scary'. Use a mirror and/or work with a partner(s) so you can feed back to each other. How will you know you are fluent? Colleagues can give you feedback, and you can use the camera on your phone to test yourself. For you, this will become an everyday skill.

4 **Practise with everyone you meet**. Go as far with a test as you can. If, for example, you only get as far as eliciting a time when someone was afraid, that is fine. This kind of practice extends how far you can go and makes you smoother and more effective. Develop your testing skills however your life permits.

5 **If you are not a Water CF, the following is an instructive experiment**. It is best to do this with a partner. Imagine something that you would be frightened of (this may be a challenge); enter it as if it was a real possibility and see what you would be seeing, hear what you would be hearing and deliberately notice how your body feels. Take care and proceed with caution. Come out, shake yourself until you feel back to normal and consider what happened to your body. Note your body sensations when undergoing fear. If you can, write down your body sensations accompanying fear, then refer to the tables in Chapter 6, beginning with Wood/anger on page 41.

6 **Pick an exercise** where you sense you have a **weakness or deficiency**. That has always been a principle of mine: not to improve your strengths, but to strengthen what you know are less-than strengths.

Summary for Water

- Find and make a list of situations where **people feel threatened** or **experience fear**.

- Notice through observation how to determine whether patients you encounter are **already expressing fear** or **seem confident and devoid of fear.**

- Ideally, work with a companion(s) in learning how to express **fear on your face**.

- Similarly, learn how to express a **groan in your voice**. Feedback is important as it enables you to learn faster. Best of all, work on the face and voice together.

- In your everyday world, be alert for the **expression of fear** and, where possible, remember and talk about **when people feel safer** and **when they feel fearful**, for example: 'What is the worst that...' and: 'How will you know the "issue" has disappeared?'.

- Be aware that **Water CFs who have lack of fear** are often missed initially.

- Experiment with feeling your body when you experience fear.

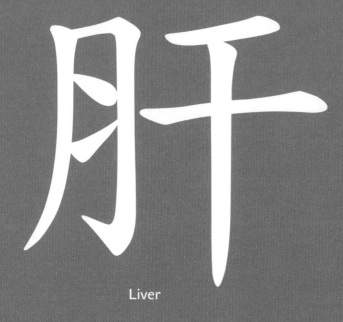

Liver

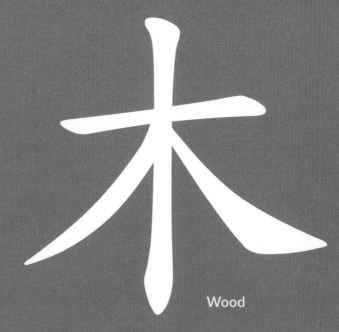

Wood

12

Testing Wood

'Anybody can become angry – that is easy, but to be
angry with the right person and to the right degree
and at the right time and for the right purpose and
in the right way – that is not within everybody's
power and is not easy.'

Aristotle

'An acorn knows how to become an oak tree –
without thought, difficult decisions or coaching –
it just knows. It has vegetation *hun*. Humans
also have *hun*, but unlike oak trees require some
external support, education and direction. The
spirit of the Wood, the *hun*, is the arbiter, recipient
and beneficiary of that external direction. Healthy
hun seeks, judges and decides on what external
support to follow.'

Anon

The emotions for Wood

Our culture lacks clarity as to when anger is appropriate or inappropriate.
In Chinese medicine this distinction is crucial and needs to be understood
via the spirit of the Wood Element.

The spirit of Wood is the *hun*. The *hun* is one's
ultimate purpose, what it is for a person to flourish.
For example, the acorn's purpose is to become
an oak tree, a human's is to grow and develop
in body, mind and spirit.[28] So, the possibilities

are enormous. As we age, we can always be asking: what is appropriate growth for our bodies, our minds and our spirits? These activities/ questions are ongoing and the world's religions and belief systems provide endless guidance and advice.

Contacting your *hun* is being in touch with your essence: what is essential for my body, my mind and my spirit? People pursue this issue in multiple ways. Humans are more complex than acorns, but the process is similar. What is human, unlike an acorn, is that man's possibilities are much more complex.

This is the function of Wood. Wood energy fuels these questions, plans and decisions and helps give us both flexibility and a sense of purpose. When a person's growth and development are frustrated, the English word anger is not quite right. What is needed is assertion, a plan and action – an outgoing push of energy – the job of healthy Wood energy.

The setting up criteria

The initial stage of testing anger is knowing how to elicit a complaint or frustration from the patient. When we are frustrated, our Wood energy comes into play. We test Wood by testing how flexible the patient is: overly flexible, just right, or inflexible?

Initiate this by asking: 'Is everything perfect?' People will often answer: 'No, of course not'. The practitioner then has an opportunity to enquire what is not perfect (maybe even 'frustrating') and there is access to material for testing Wood. Another way we can do this is that we develop an ear for conflict, especially when we hear that a patient may be suffering from another's behaviour.

Then we use the setting up criteria. These are the guidelines for testing anger. They are not exact, but their purpose is to give you a sense of what must be in place to carry out the test and your judgement will, over time, become more precise.

For Wood, the setting up criteria are:
- there is an **abuse** the patient has suffered
- there must be an **abuser**, which can't be God, but can be an organisation, for instance Network Rail, that someone can rightfully be angry at, or a person who the patient believes has wronged them
- the abuse is **recent** or **ongoing**; it is best that it is not too far in the past
- there is some **wrongness**, where wrongness is defined either as illegal or by convention unfair, inappropriate, or something in your culture

that is not considered fair, just, or appropriate – this can be subtle, especially in a multicultural world.

Once we discover an item of unjust frustration, we can, as emotion testers, express anger on the patient's behalf and ask the patient to respond.

Recognising anger on the face

How do we know that our patient is angry and to what degree? On the face, anger manifests as:

- eyes become hard and staring
- eyebrows come closer together
- lower eyelids get tight
- lips are tight, tense or twitchy.

These are the 'parts' of anger and as practitioners we need to learn to recognise the many degrees of expression – from **slight annoyance** to **full blown rage**.

Slight annoyance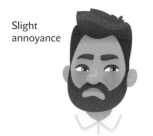

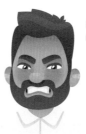 Full blown rage

Why does treatment on the Wood Element help a Wood CF?

A Wood CF, being prone to anger or its suppression, undergoes bodily tension. For a description of this, revisit the details of 'Bodily sensations associated with feeling angry' in Chapter 6, page 41. Treatment of someone who is a Wood CF lessens the occurrence of these and this is usually the basis of the Wood CF's claim to be feeling 'better in myself'. If the Wood CF occurs more from Blood deficiency, this may be less true.

Testing anger

Parking your car across a neighbour's driveway and blocking access for several hours may not be illegal, but there is something wrong about it. You do, of course need to know a culture to judge wrongness.

What? You mean this person blocked your driveway for **four** hours?

As an example of a test, assume that access to your driveway is blocked by a carelessly parked car. You are frustrated. There seems to be no other spaces and you have things to do. Access to your driveway is suddenly important.

In sympathy with the patient, your words as a practitioner might be: 'What? You mean this person blocked your driveway for four hours?'. This needs to be said with the beginnings of some anger including some 'shout' in the voice. Shout, the English translation of *hu*, does not necessarily mean 'loud'. It means the inclusion of emphasis on specific syllables, as we do when we are angry. Here it is again, with the emphasis shown in bold: '**What**? You mean this person **blocked** your driveway for **four** hours? You must have been really **annoyed**!'. The *hu* is not necessarily loud, but certain words have emphasis. The flow is not smooth.

In addition, you make it clear, by pointing at the imaginary abuser, that your anger is *at the abuser* and definitely *not* at the patient. You are leading them and asking them to follow. How the patient responds can be classified as:

- a **normal response**, an expression of an appropriate level of anger at the abuser
- a **verbal denial** of anger, but with signs of anger on the face, what we might call lack of anger or denied anger, or
- an **excess response** (excessive anger).

The last two above suggest the person may be a Wood CF. The denial of anger with anger signs on the face can be described as a lack of anger, or maybe a lack of appropriate assertion; the person saying they are not angry, but at the same time showing signs that they are angry, specifically, a tight mouth, hard eyes and *hu* (a shout) in the voice. These signs may be subtle, chronic or both.

You must have been really annoyed

That is the essence of an anger test. It takes time and patience interacting with people in this way to begin to trust your judgement about the appropriateness or otherwise of the response. Be sensitive, and careful to take into account reponses arising from different cultural backgrounds.

First you need to learn to be **expressive to just the right degree** and **second** you learn how, *at the same time*, to **observe and judge the response** – initially a difficult combination. On occasions, the response's appropriateness or otherwise will be obvious and that makes the learning easier. For example, the person looks startled as if to say: 'You expect me to be angry? No way! I don't do anger!'. Or, they get angry to an excessive degree. It is practise, practise and more practise, until the norms and the abnormal responses become obvious.

There are some variations. Without any test, you may see signs of anger on the face and hear a shout in the voice, but the person denies being angry. Alternatively, it is as if they sense you coming and the test just never seems to come to fruition. You think you have heard an abuse, there seems to be a wrong, which is recent or ongoing, but when you invite anger to arise, the patient denies it and goes blank – signs of an unwillingness to show anger. They are responding with a lack of anger and we need to be practised enough to slip behind their protection, or read the disconnect.

Or, the patient may manifest anger from the start. This anger in your judgement is excessive and inappropriate given the context. In this case, there is no need to elicit anger; it is just there, excess, blatant and in your judgement inappropriate. No need for a test. The more you have tested Wood, the easier it will be to make such judgements. Observation and/ or the testing of anger is an art form nourished and developed by paying close attention, and practise.

Examples of recognising anger

I remember a patient from my early practice. His name was Mike and he would come into the clinic in a wheelchair. He seemed permanently angry and would shout at the carer who brought him as if she were stupid and abusing him, whereas the reverse seemed obvious. His wheelchair, which he controlled, would force others out of the way. His voice was shouting and very harsh. There was no need for a test; he was obviously inappropriately angry. If anger occurred on a scale of 1 to 10, he seemed to be continuously on 10. He appeared, just from observation, with no interaction, to be expressing excessive anger.

Often, these indicators become subtle, chronic. Recently, on a train journey, a couple sat opposite me, took out books and began to read. I was observing their faces: both of their mouths were tense and twitchy, their lower eyelids seemed tense and their eyes hard. Such observations are tricky because they usually presuppose a norm and a change: a tense mouth is compared with a relaxed mouth, tight lower eyelids are compared with relaxed ones and hard eyes are compared with soft eyes. So, to look for the first time and judge someone's mouth to be tense or eyes to be hard requires enough previous observations to recognise a mouth which is tense but could be more relaxed, and similarly with the eyes.

With this couple, after five minutes, there was a spoken interchange: both spoke in voices that were quiet, but nevertheless contained a shout. They were clearly comfortable with each other, but my observations strongly suggested that they were both Wood CFs. She was pale, dull; he was green around the mouth. They were manifesting **chronics** on their faces.

Another patient in the early days of my practice baffled me. Susie was gentle, fortyish, self-effacing and reminded me of a tame mouse. She had no emphasis in the voice, she was extremely gentle, and her complaint was pain. I asked JR Worsley for help and within two minutes he took me outside the treatment room and said she was a Wood CF. I had missed the absence of any shout in the voice, tension in the area of the eyes or tension in the mouth area. That gets labelled lack of anger.

Another lady, Alice was in her 40s and suffering from increasing numbness of one leg (to the extent that she had begun falling down). She described how a doctor had told her, after various tests, that there was nothing wrong with her and that she should go home and forget about her complaint. Having carefully clarified the details and what had been said to her, I entered a mild state of anger and pointing (as if at the consultant) I said: 'You must have been angry at him'. She suddenly withdrew into herself and said, very quietly: 'Well, no, I just took it on the chin' and she looked away. She was a Wood CF and treatment helped immensely. There are different ways to be a Wood CF.

Finally, Cynthia, another 40-year-old female patient said that she needed courage to leave her husband. That was her main complaint. She was a Wood CF and I remembered the timidity of the Gall Bladder and was thinking she needed courage to decide. I assumed she would get that and leave her husband. After five treatments, I asked about the situation at home and she said: 'That's sorted. I have made the decision to stay and feel very good about that.' A learning for me: balance the patient's energy and let the balance do its work.

Wood self-training tasks

1 **Make a list of 15 common occurrences where people are frustrated and might get angry**. For example, you get a bill for something you didn't receive; someone carelessly bumps into you in a shopping mall; a train is late and you missed the beginning of an exam; a promised and important delivery, for which you remained home, doesn't turn up; your child has promised something for the fifth time and not delivered; you have been on holiday and on return you find your house/ flat has been burgled; a colleague at work tells fibs behind your back; you break down on the motorway and the breakdown service promises to be there in 20 minutes, and after 90 minutes still hasn't arrived.

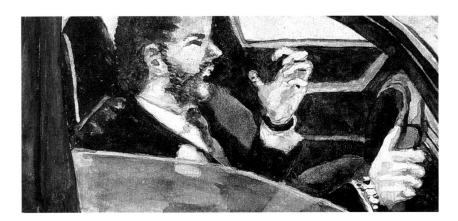

2 When you have the list, **run each through the who/abuse/angry filter**; do they meet the criteria?

3 **Work on your voice: both the tone of voice and the words people use when they are angry**. Ideally, if you can, do these exercises with a colleague or in a group. Why? 'Feedback is the Breakfast of Champions'.[29] You will learn much quicker when receiving feedback. Think of real statements you can make when you feel anger and use them. Think of people/organisations in the world with whom you strongly disagree. Take phrases like 'I think you are greedy and irresponsible' or 'They did what?' and say them out loud. Put emphasis on the right syllables so that if anyone heard you, they would know you are angry. Make a scale from 1 to 5 where 1 is 'a little angry' and 5 is 'very angry'. Do a 1, then a 2, then a 3, then a 4 and finally a 5. Do this with a colleague enough times to develop 'expressive flexibility' with the sound of anger. Get and give feedback, even on the phone. Make it enjoyable. Review regularly until vocal fluency with anger is yours.

4 **You might think this is artificial, because you are not genuinely angry**. But, it is normal to be angry on others' behalf, is it not? For example, parents easily get angry at someone abusing their children, or a person can be angry at someone abusing their partner. Or, we get angry at hearing how the dictator in another country is abusing their citizens. So, you can do this for a patient.

5 **Learn to look angry whilst producing an angry voice**, so others would look at you and know instantly you are angry. (This may have already occurred naturally in point 3 above.) How?
   – Harden your eyes, let your eyebrows pull together
   – Tense your lower eyelids
   – Make your lips be tight, tense or twitchy
Remember, you do this *on behalf of the patient,* directing it at the transgressor, never *at* the patient. Use a mirror and involve your face and body. At the same time, bring in the angry voice and spit out the words. Get to the stage that you can easily express anger on your face and in your body. Line up your imaginary transgressors and rail at them full blast. Visualise these people and give them 'what for', with passion. Having done this on your own or ideally with colleagues, learn to regulate your expression, (as we did previously with the voice), for example, let 1 be a 'little annoyed' and 5 be 'very annoyed', choose your words and do a 1 to 5 and then 5 back down to 1.

Regard this as practise just like a musician practising scales. Enjoy it. It won't harm you and it will make you a better emotion tester.

6 **Get a study buddy** for the exercises and/or for demonstrating your new skills. Swap experiences. Ideally, work with others on all of the above exercises. Your learning will be faster and more thorough.

7 **Learn the bodily sensations of anger** Deliberately remember a time(s) when you were mildly annoyed. Focus first on what annoyed you; then focus on the accompanying bodily sensations. (Revisit 'Bodily sensations associated with feeling angry' in Chapter 6, page 41.) Notice what you do internally when angry.

8 **Pick a task** where you sense you have a **weakness or deficiency** and feel you might enjoy **developing skills**. That has always been a principle of mine: not to improve your strengths, but to strengthen what you know are your weaknesses, especially when you will enjoy the process and benefit from your own greater flexibility.

Summary for Wood

- Be aware that both **anger** and **no anger** can be **appropriate** or **inappropriate**.

- Find complaints where the patient was not treated fairly, where there is a **who**, an **abuse** and the event is **recent** or **ongoing**.

- Learn to express **increasing levels of anger,** both on your **face** and in your **voice**.

- Be sure that you indicate the who to be angry at is **not the patient, but the apparent transgressor/offender**.

- Judge the **level of anger** (via voice, face and gesture) to be appropriate or not.

- When you feel anger, rather than focusing on what you are angry at or about, notice the **sensations in your body**.

In the next chapter, you will find an exercise titled 'Slow-motion emotion testing' that enables you to learn the testing skills in comfort.

13

Slow-motion emotion testing

'Stare at who you want to become'
'Steal without apology'
'Be willing to be stupid'
'Don't fall for the prodigy myth'

Daniel Coyle, *The Little Book of Talent*

Learning how to emotion test

Slow-motion emotion testing is a basic exercise for learning how to emotion test. It can be used by anyone, from beginners to practitioners to teachers. Learning to test and refining your skills is an ongoing, career-long process.

Emotion testing is the process of interacting with a patient so that each of the Five Elements is visited emotionally with the purpose of assessing whether the emotion of that Element is **in balance** or **out of balance**. For example, if the Fire Element is out of balance, the resonating emotions – joy/sadness – will show **excess** or **deficiency**. This is the essence of emotion testing.

The process appears initially to be subtle or complicated. It does take application to learn it, but so did walking, discriminating colours or speaking and writing, although as adults we simply take those skills for granted. In addition, and this is a personal opinion, learning to emotion test has benefits outside as well as inside the treatment room. It helps a lot in everyday life.

What are the components of the exercise? You need at least six or seven participants, but the process can accommodate 30 to 35, possibly more. The exercise can be done in a class, study group or anywhere folks who want to learn can gather. It can be adapted to suit the skill level of the learners.

Assume we have a group of around 20. The room is set up like a classroom, with the teacher or group leader/organiser at the front and two chairs (preferably high ones), one for the person testing (the **emotion tester** in the role of **practitioner**) and another for the person being tested (the **testee** acting as the **patient**).

The job of the emotion tester

- Gaining rapport
- Knowing the process of the various tests
- Setting up a test by evoking specific content on the stage of the patient's (testee's) mind
- Delivering, with the right expression, a request either to express or to take in some emotion
- Observing the nature of the response
- Judging the 'normality/abnormality' of the response

Several skills must be developed and used together (or in sequence) and, like juggling, giving a talk or learning to drive a car, this requires learning one part of the process at a time.

Slow-motion emotion testing is an ideal answer, because the learner, whenever they feel uncertain where to go, can simply stop, ask for help and elicit several suggestions from fellow learners who have been watching, but with *no pressure to perform*.[30] The practice is made easy and skills grow.

The slow-motion emotion testing process

With a new group, the group leader initiates the process by acting as the emotion tester; this is not necessary in an experienced group.

To start the process the **emotion tester** (acting as the practitioner):
- interacts briefly with the **testee** (acting as patient)
- experiences some uncertainty
- explains to the testee that they are going to seek help from the main group
- asks the group for help; what to do next
- gets several opinions
- chooses one of the options
- returns to the testee, and continues in the same vein.

During the interchange between emotion tester and main group, the testee can listen, but does not take part and the main group does not interact with the testee. *This is an important rule*: the main group does not interact with the person being tested, and vice versa.

The emotion tester considers the group's suggestions, thanks them, turns back to the person being tested and engages again. The process is now set in motion. The emotion tester tests, and at any moment of hesitation, stops and turns to the main group for help. For example, the advice might be:

- **persist** with the current Element test, or
- **go to another** Element, and
- **how to get there** (specifying the exact words).

This 'stop and start again' may happen several times. Any one incident raised by the emotion tester can lead to tests for two or three Elements. There is no specific 'right' order in which Elements can be tested.

Everyone needs to embrace the idea that there may be dead ends, but no 'mistakes'. It is also important to understand that this exercise is *not* for clinical use. The group leader should ensure that it does not turn into a dispute about CFs, and no one's CF should be confirmed.

At some point the person leading the group says: 'Stop', and gives positive feedback, telling the emotion tester how well they did and reinforcing/articulating any good practice or learning/good testing that was observed. Then the emotion tester steps down and rejoins the main group. The testee becomes the emotion tester and a new person becomes the testee. Depending on the enthusiasm of the group, the group leader can ask for a volunteer, or move to the next person in line (back row, front row, whatever) making sure that it doesn't become a 'shall I, shan't I?' process.

How long does the emotion tester get? This can be determined by the group leader, five minutes could be the norm, but also consider how many are in attendance, how much learning is occurring (remember the main group is learning as well as the emotion testers) and the time available. Throughout, the person leading the group relies on their judgement as to how things are going and adjusts accordingly.

This exercise will accelerate the process of learning how to emotion test. Here is a summary of the roles and interactions between group members.

Slow-motion emotion testing: roles and interactions

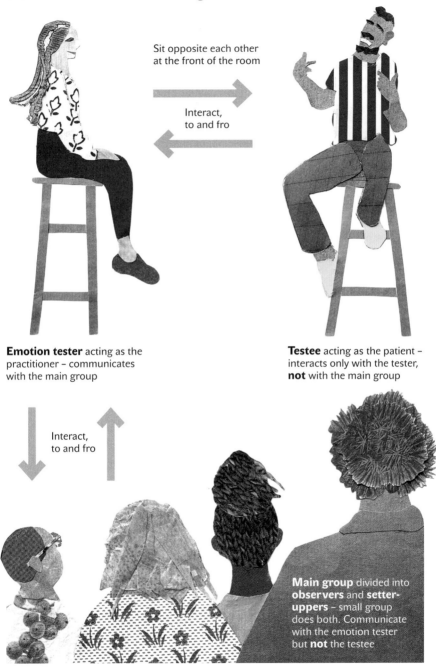

Sit opposite each other at the front of the room

Interact, to and fro

Emotion tester acting as the practitioner – communicates with the main group

Testee acting as the patient – interacts only with the tester, **not** with the main group

Interact, to and fro

Main group divided into **observers** and **setter-uppers** – small group does both. Communicate with the emotion tester but **not** the testee

Emotion tester (practitioner)

- Shouldn't feel pressured, or let themself get stuck – can always stop and go back to the group for next step
- Invites the group to make suggestions – specifically about which Element, and what to say
- Listens, appreciates the feedback and decides for themself how to proceed
- Always asks the testee's permission to stop and start, and thanks the main group for suggestions
- Says 'hello' to restart with the testee

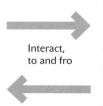

Interact, to and fro

Testee (patient)

- Responds normally
- Talks only to the emotion tester
- Does **not** talk or interact with the main group

Group leader/teacher

- States the rules clearly
- Takes the first turn as emotion tester, if the group is new
- Determines when a tester's turn is over, and who goes next
- Keeps everyone in role, if necessary
- Puts learnings into words for learners
- Encourages the tester and makes sure they are not concerned about making 'mistakes'
- Sets the tone, and helps make the process pleasurable for all
- Makes sure that the process does not turn into a dispute about CFs

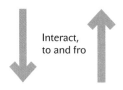

Interact, to and fro

Main group

Minimum group size is 6 or 7. Groups of 16+ can be split by function: **observers** say what has happened and **setter-uppers** suggest where to go next. If less than 16, the main group does both.

Observers

- Only communicate with the emotion tester
- Notice significant changes in the face, breathing, bodily movement or voice
- When the testee is being tested, judge whether they are taking it in, and expressing appropriately

Setter-uppers

- Only communicate with the emotion tester
- Track the setting up
- Notice how the tester's words direct the testee
- Listen for useful and less useful words or phrases
- Words that are 'delivery' (see page 55)
- Stay aware of what has been learned already
- Help the testee decide where to go next, and what specific words are needed to get there

14

Developing touch to express

Touch can be used to feel pulses, temperature, the location of points, the body's propensity to retain water and more. Touch is for collecting this information. Alternatively, can touch be used to express?

When testing, to express an emotion, we can use our:
- **face**
- **voice**, and
- our **choice of words**.

When we test emotions, we can also use **touch**. Early on, I was with a new patient and a colleague was with me. We often went in with each other's patients. I was about to take pulses, standing beside the couch, holding the patient's hand. I had given the patient sympathy and was ready to take pulses but kept expressing sympathy through my hand. The patient was an Earth CF and became very uncomfortable with tears welling up. My colleague nudged me and indicated with a head nod that we should leave the room. Outside he told me that I had expressed sympathy, the patient couldn't take it in, was probably an Earth CF, and I had seemed not to have noticed and was now making the patient very uncomfortable with my continued expression of sympathy via my hand. All part of a working/learning day, except it made me wonder about using touch, not just to take in information, but to express. After that, I experimented with the nature of touch as part of a test by expressing warmth, sympathy/understanding/support, respect, reassurance, or resoluteness. You should not take this too seriously, but you may want to experiment with the following exercise.

Experimenting with touch as expression

With two people, **A** is the receiver and **B** is the sender.

- **A** sits in a chair, lays their arm on the armrest and closes their eyes.

- **B** sits or stands beside **A** so as to be able to lay a hand on **A**'s forearm, or holds **A**'s hand as if taking pulses.

- **B** picks two of the Five Elements and use the positive expression for each, that is: joy (Fire), sympathy/understanding/support (Earth), a positive inner quality, or PIQ (Metal), reassurance (Water) or resoluteness/firmness (Wood). I would suggest starting with sympathy/ understanding/support (Earth) and resoluteness/firmness (Wood), because they will possibly contrast more.

- **A** knows that, via **B**'s hand they will feel, for example, either resoluteness/firmness (Wood) or sympathy/understanding/support (Earth).

- **B** then chooses one of these emotions, accesses the feeling within her/ himself, and lays a hand on **A**'s forearm or holds the hand as if taking pulses, either for five seconds.

- **B** records the feeling they felt, either resoluteness/firmness or sympathy/understanding/support

- **B** then accesses the other feeling, and either with their hand on the arm or as if taking pulses, expresses the other feeling. **A** will feel a difference and labels the two the best they can.

- **B** then describes to **A** what they were trying communicate, first and then second.

- When you achieve some success, either add another emotion or choose a different pair. Enjoy!

Now try this – it is really an extension of expressing any of the positive feelings described above. You enter the emotion (probably feeling it in your face and chest) and let the feeling spread to include your arms and hands. This may seem easy and may seem difficult.

It seems to me we are all in the same boat, having some sort of choice between suffering the negative emotions of our CF or reducing these and working towards positive ones. Herein lies the beauty of Five Element constitutional acupuncture:
- more **joy** and less **sadness**
- more **balanced connection** to others and less **confusion** as to whose needs are in the foreground
- more **connection to our spiritual side** and less to **our wants**
- less driven by **fear** and more by an **appropriate sense of courage**, and
- less **confusion** about how to act and more **internal direction**.

15

The rich rewards of knowing the constitutional factor (CF)

This book has covered several, although not all, aspects of Five Element acupuncture diagnosis. Sometimes treatment blocks take precedence. And sometimes clearing pathogens may be necessary. But a major part of the job is finding the CF and that has been the focus.

1 Finding the patient's constitutional type is an important step towards getting the best possible changes from treatment. See research by Jackie Shaw and others.[31]

2 Improving the patient's Five Element imbalance, for most patients, is the quickest way to achieve both short- and long-term benefits. Much of what patients bring to practitioners has arisen from their original Elemental imbalance spreading via the energetic cycles.

3 Discovering the CF imbalance is predominantly a sensory activity, based on seeing patients' facial colour, hearing an inappropriate sound in their voices, smelling their predominant body odours and through emotion testing, discovering their most out-of-balance Five Element emotion.

4 You might think it couldn't be simpler. But, as it turns out, developing/ enlarging our sensory capabilities takes effort, and an effort which is often puzzling. Why? We tend to believe that we can already see, hear, smell, and recognise emotions. We can, but the relevant depth of sensory acuity is not necessarily a given. JR Worsley convinced me of this by demonstrating his near impeccable ability to diagnose CFs. The only response was continuing sensory refinement.

5 Habits of perception become unconscious and, we rarely notice how conditioned and repetitive we are. Changing sensory habits requires a consistent effort and finding ways to practise.

6 This effort is best done both on one's own and with others: on one's own, to overcome our individual and habitual patterns of perception; with others, to get agreement, accuracy and a common language. Such a language uses words based both in the use of our senses and multiple comparisons with others' sensing.

7 When assessing patients' progress, we have two sources of feedback: patient reports and our own senses. We keep these separate but use them both for assessing how a patient is progressing. It is a challenge when, on occasions, they don't agree.

8 The rewards of this process, first for patients and second for practitioners can be amazing.

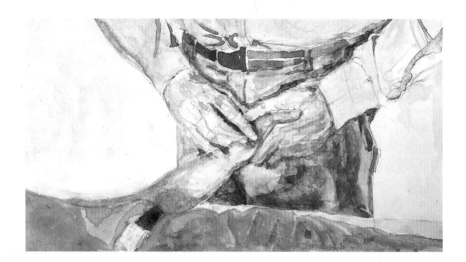

Appendix: Advanced rapport-building skills

Advanced matching skills

I saw no evidence in China of our doctor, Dr Li, matching patients. Doing excellent TCM does not, I believe, require matching skills – rather, observation skills. As an example, my doctor in China enjoyed teaching us. One clinic session he was observing the line-up of patients and I sensed he was getting excited. It turned out that he noticed from his notes two older patients with the same complaint waiting on a row of chairs, both female; both with asthma, but one large and overweight and the other, skinny and frail. Same complaint, different diagnosis. Time for him to teach, which he did with gusto. One was Kidney *yin* deficient, the other Kidney *yang* deficient. His visual acuity was superb, his teacher excitement endearing and his diagnosis spot on. He required no matching; his eyes did the work.

So, why match so thoroughly? Dr Li had many years of experience and was considered, in China, good enough to teach foreigners. He was a good example of how well you can use TCM. And he had around 35 years' experience. He did not diagnose CFs. At CICM we teach CFs *and* TCM. The challenge for the student lies in whether to place emphasis on TCM or on Five Element skills. Both are best to learn, but at some time a choice may emerge, which can be made consciously.

Those who choose to become excellent Five Element diagnosticians need primarily to develop their sensory and rapport skills first and, at the same time, know how to look up differentiations of their patients' complaints. Those who choose to be excellent TCM diagnosticians need to know their differentiations and let their sensory acuity grow naturally in the clinic. I believe there is a choice, even though my choice should be obvious.

Back in Chapter 2 we looked at three fundamental aspects of matching to achieve strong rapport: **tempo**, **posture** and the **voice**.

In this appendix we focus on other, more advanced matching skills. Here is a reminder of the table of matching options:

Matching	Direct	Adjusting	Examples
*Matchings that **don't** require timing*			
Tempo of: • speech • movement • thinking *See page 24*	Adjust to patient's tempo in three ways, one at a time. Speech/thinking will be close	Easier to slow than speed up. Can be frustrating and hard to do	Very slow speech; agitated movements; a mind which makes quick leaps
Posture *See page 25*	Become closer to patient's posture	Forwards/ backwards; erect/slumped	Degrees of accuracy from gross to subtle
Voice *See page 25*	Five Element sound becomes closer to that of patient's	Based on Five Element sounds	An Earth CF practitioner puts 'shout' into their voice
Breathing	Match rate and area (chest, Middle, or Lower Burner)	Can be quite exact	Easiest done when holding a hand – just after/whilst pulse taking
*Matchings that **do** require timing*			
Key gestures	**Indirect** 'Integrated into' practitioner's behaviour at appropriate moments	Often the arms/ hands/face	Cutting with edge of hand; palms upwards with eyes wide open
Key words	'Fitted into' what practitioner says	Both word(s) and tone	Spoken as if it's my word. May accompany gestures
Sensory predicates *See page 121*	Notice visual/auditory/ tactile/kinaesthetic words/bias and take these on yourself	You need the flexibility/practise to do this	Patient talks mainly about what they see and practitioner then matches

Matching all aspects is a massive task and you do *not* have to match everything. Over time you will be able to answer the question: 'Do I have enough rapport to proceed?', remembering that good rapport enables emotion testing, improves CF diagnosis, and encourages the patient to continue with treatment. Let's take a closer look at matching **key gestures** and **key words**.

Matching key gestures

Gestures, unlike posture, are brief and thus need to be noticed, assessed and then introduced at appropriate moments in the flow of your own behaviour. **Firstly**, practise involves **watching people and paying attention to their gestures**. What do they do with their hands/arms and sometimes with their facial expressions – especially when they are talking? It is a movement that is 'part' of what they are saying. A **key gesture** is one which is both repeated and seems to carry feeling with it.

Secondly, consider, were you in conversation with them, how you could **introduce a similar gesture into your behaviour** *as if it were yours*. Do not mimic them; notice it and replicate it, but make it your own.

An example of **gesture matching** convinced me of its efficacy. I saw a patient for a colleague. As we talked, I noticed that the patient's glasses kept slipping down his nose and he would push them back in place with his right index finger. As it happened, my glasses also slipped down my nose, not as much and I simply left them there. I started using my right index finger, at intervals, *my* intervals, to return my glasses further up my nose. When we finished the conversation, the patient told me that he was most grateful and it was one of the most interesting conversations he had ever had and he thanked me profusely. The conversation was not particularly interesting, and I can think of many reasons why he said what he did – just being polite or wanting to express appreciation. But I was sure it was the finger pushing my glasses up my nose. Don't believe me; experiment.

The first learning stage is to just to observe, to notice what people do. Decide what counts as a gesture. It must be repetitive and must be an expression of feeling. What then? You incorporate it into your behaviour in a manner similar to how the patient incorporates it into his/her behaviour. This is not a direct match, but an **indirect match**. Practise in groups, in cafés or watching TV.

Matching key words

When talking we use a smaller vocabulary than the one we possess. We tend to overuse certain words, repeating them with feeling. Listen for repeated words that also seem to have emotion built into them.

For example, a patient used to describe his life as a series of conflicts with people he referred to as 'the so-and-sos'. I managed almost teasingly to refer to some new people he mentioned as 'so-and-sos' and he was surprised and laughed heartily. It was both a conscious and unconscious moment, but it led to greater rapport. I would say he definitely felt that I understood him.

There are many matching possibilities. Consider first what is easy and effective, with an emphasis on easy. Practise and evaluate your results. Learning to match can be very enjoyable for us and rewarding for those we match. It brings us closer together.

Empty matching

Matching usually involves a decision to match something specific and then carrying out the match. Empty matching is a more refined skill, to be done after you have some experience of ordinary matching. It involves waiting for an expression and immediately – no conscious thought – you match the expression spontaneously. You may do this already when you meet an old friend, and you match their pleasure at meeting you with yours at meeting them. This matching happens naturally. But you can also do it deliberately.

Whatever the 'state' of the person, you match it – immediately and spontaneously. If they are **glum**, you respond, no thought, with glum. If they seem **confused**, you respond, no thought, with confused. If they are **excited**, you respond, no thought, with excited. Unlike the matching already discussed, there is no conscious decision about what to match. It is worth repeating that you very likely do this already when it is easy and occurs naturally. The difference here is that you are extending your range: you match whatever appears.

> **To recap** You decide *beforehand* that whatever the person's state, you will match it and then do it. *Match spontaneously, but with care.* It is, of course, necessary to have matched consciously before attempting this exercise because it will challenge your flexibility. This will be a development of the matching skills already developed. Use the following exercise.

Experimenting with empty matching to develop spontaneous matching skills

1 Form a group of three, **A**, **B** and **C** where **A** is the **expresser**, **B** the **matcher** and **C** the **observer**.

2 If **B** is on **A**'s right, **A** turns to his/her left and accesses a feeling, for example, feeling angry about some issue, pleased about something, or maybe sad – the clearer and stronger the feeling, the better. This should take no more than seven seconds.

3 **A** then turns to **B** and expresses the feeling both in words and non-verbally. **A** uses no more than ten words and makes the facial expression clear. **A** then stops. This expression of words and face should take a maximum of three to seven seconds. **C** can be manager, making sure that the time constraints are followed.

4 **B** responds immediately, matching **A**'s state. **B** does *not* ask a question; **B** just expresses. This is **empty matching** – you are learning to match directly *without* any content or need to 'understand'.

5 **A** then labels the match as a **hit**, **miss** or **almost**. In my experience this labelling is understood quickly by practically all participants.

6 Depending on the judgement:
  – If it is a **hit**, switch roles and rotate: **A** becomes **B** becomes **C**.
  – If it is a **miss**, **A** or **C** can give feedback as to what wasn't right – *if they can*. And in the same roles, **A**, **B** and **C** have one more try. Then rotate.
  – If it is an **almost**, then **A** attempts to explain why, for example what was or wasn't there which made the response an almost. **B** then gets a second attempt, bearing in mind that **A**'s expression may not be quite the same as before. Then rotate.
  – You are not making a judgement about success. The person expressing may well express something simple or mixed and make **A**'s job easy or more difficult.

7 It may take a few attempts, before learners stop giggling and recognise the exercise's learning potential. For many learners, what gets in the way is the feeling that, before they can match, they need to understand. You don't. Just match.

Neuro-linguistic programming (NLP) and chunking

The remainder of this appendix draws on ideas from NLP, which has influenced and fed into my Chinese medicine practice and teaching for many years. Students, with a few exceptions, tend not to have the time to develop such skills and the exam system favours book learning. I learned in a different context, but include these insights for completeness. These are advanced skills which will enrich your understanding of rapport.

This section relates back to the rapport example of the biker and his female practitioner, where what they had in common was wanting to 'look good' (page 18) and to the example of the Welsh practitioner and her patient who seemed concerned about money when he was actually concerned about family (page 19). The intention is to clarify the NLP terms **chunking up** and **chunking down**. Understanding them can lead to a greater degree of flexibility and much better rapport.

The nouns we use are of varying degrees of abstraction. For example, the word 'furniture' covers things like sofas, chairs, tables, and big cushions. Any one of these, for example, 'chairs', covers a wide variety of chairs: kitchen chairs, folding chairs, office chairs and so on. Those are examples of chunking down.

Going in the reverse direction is chunking up. We could go up from a stool in the pantry to kitchen furniture to domestic furniture to furniture in general to 'goods and chattels' or whatever. Flexible thinking requires chunking in both directions, up and down, and it is useful to remember that different people chunk differently: we often chunk in similar ways, but not always. The key message is that chunking up can help in the search for similarity and rapport.

Back to the biker and his practitioner. Different genders, different contexts, but what they valued in common was 'looking good'. Similarly, the practitioner from Wales asked her patient to chunk up and found they shared the importance of family. Chunking up is often a direct path to what we have in common.

To summarise, a core question is: 'What is important about X, where X is something that the person invests time/attention in'? This can be varied to suit the context, by varying the words:
- What is it about X that you enjoy?
- You really enjoy that. What matters about X?
- You spend time on that. What's important about that?
- Why is X important to you?

Suppose you don't like smoking and a patient does. Ask them what they like about smoking. They will say something like: 'It's relaxing'. You might agree with relaxing. Within one person, values, like relaxing occur in hierarchies. Someone may seem obsessed about money, but when you investigate, what is important about money is 'providing for my family'. Then you can ask: 'What is important about providing for your family?' At this point, people often pause, as if the first answer, family, was just so basic, they don't know what to say. Make contact on the level of family, not money or what you saw as meanness.

If you don't like something about someone, ask them: 'What's important to you about that?' Wait to be surprised. Most people (probably all) at their core are likeable. Find what is likeable and share it. Build rapport.

Utilising representational (rep) systems and choosing a state

Neuro-linguistic programming draws attention to what are called **sensory predicates**. These are words we use which give a clue to the sense you are using internally when thinking or re-presenting the world to yourself, for example:

- replaying this morning's meeting (past)
- going over a future conversation with a friend (future)
- wondering what the holiday will be like (future)
- remembering how it used to be before so-and-so died (past)
- trying to decide what you need to do today (future)
- remembering where you left your glasses (past).

We can do any of these using a mix of internal pictures, words, sounds, feelings and sometimes maybe even tastes and smells. NLP calls these **representational systems** or **rep systems** for short, because we are re-presenting previous or future experience to ourselves in order to daydream, plan, decide, reflect, puzzle or calculate. People have sensory preferences as to how they do this:

- a painter may often think more in visual images
- a musician more in sounds
- a lawyer in words (called auditory digital)
- a sculptor in bodily feelings/sensations.

I once saw a conductor being interviewed who was explaining how he could hear several different groups of instruments contributing to the overall sound of the orchestra. I would have happily traded ears with him, but then I wondered about his sight and bodily sensations. We often develop one sense over others, and this may derive from our natural talents, upbringing, jobs or learned skills.

Matching rep systems is a step too far for most acupuncturists because it requires more attention and effort than matching generally. So look on it as an advanced skill.

Our inner worlds are not on display, but they can be assessed in two ways:

1 Listening to the person's use of **sensory words**

2 Observing a person's **eye accessing cues**

We will start with a person's **sensory predicates**, or **words**. We can listen to a person's words for the sense they imply, for example:

- **visual** – words like red, bright, clear, sparkling, show, see, and phrases like 'crystal clear', 'tunnel vision, 'see through', 'take a view'
- **kinaesthetic** – words like heavy, hard, weighty, pressure, grasp, lukewarm, gross, yuk, uncomfortable, firm, flow and phrases like 'in the groove', 'hanging in there', 'boils down to', 'get a load of this'
- **auditory tonal** – words like bark, screech, mellifluous, listen, loud, screech, grating, and phrases like 'tune in', 'clear as a bell', 'sounds like', 'purrs like a kitten'
- **auditory digital** – words like script, thoughts, interview, sequence, journey and phrases like 'due diligence', 'consider the idea', 'make sense of', or 'to sum up'.

Listening carefully to a person's language will gradually lead you to notice differences in the balance of their words and therefore their sensory preferences. You could be fairly sure that a university law professor will use more **sensory-neutral, digital** words than the first violinist in the London Symphony Orchestra who will use more **auditory sensory** words. And, the highest goal scoring professional footballer will use more **kinaesthetic** words than a painter whose vocabulary will be packed with more **visual** words.

TEDTalks are something you could watch on YouTube, determining the speaker's preferred rep system by listening out for the words they use. You would need to listen to more than one to notice differences. It is not surprising that people whose internal worlds are substantially different do not 'connect' as well as those whose internal worlds match. Rep systems make a difference to rapport.

Noticing a person's eye accessing cues is the second way of detecting a person's preferred sensory system. These cues are eye movements, for example, moving your eyes up and to the left is normally for making **remembered visual images** or moving them down and to the right is **kinaesthetic**, for accessing feelings. Initially, just watch someone on TV talking and notice how their eyes move up and down or in different directions. The diagram opposite shows the way most people's eye movements are organised.

Learning to use this information requires practise, of the following sort. I find a partner and ask a question which I am sure would make the person imagine (**construct**) a visual image, for example:

Eye accessing cues

Constructed visual

Remembered visual

Constructed auditory

Remembered auditory

Kinaesthetic (accessing feelings)

Auditory digital

'Can you imagine a horse painted red?' Then I notice where their eyes go. And so on.

There is one important proviso. Some people, especially left-handers, have the sides reversed. For example, 'remembered visual' is still up, but on the right where 'constructed visual' would be for most people.

There are two ways to assess someone's preferred representational systems: a person's language and their eye-accessing cues. No one uses only one channel, but people have natural preferences which may dictate whether they end up as a singer, copywriter, solicitor, painter or athlete. Also, training to be a solicitor or singer may influence your rep system of choice. It is all about tendencies and/or preferences.

If these differences are not intuitively obvious, do you know someone who is:
- a technical writer, a bit wired, enjoys talking, has a big vocabulary, reads abstract stuff a lot, and doesn't often express feelings, but is always good with words?
- a bit overweight, is slow both in body and speech, likes good food, casual clothes and has a high priority on being comfortable and likes to touch and hug and hangs on to your hand having shaken it, often with a two-handed handshake?
- always playing music, listens to music through headphones, likes to sing, tells stories, plays an instrument, enjoys chatting or writing.
- fussy about her clothes, likes to look good, has a quick mind, is definitely not touchy/feely and likes cinema/TV, and going to galleries?

A person's **preferred representational system** is the one that he/she uses most often to think, decide, ponder, reminisce, and so on. And yes, people will use all rep systems to some extent. To refine your rapport, match the patient's preferred sensory system.

Endnotes

1 Angela Hicks, John Hicks and Peter Mole, *Five Element Constitutional Acupuncture*, London: Churchill Livingstone, 2nd edition, 2010

2 My exploration of Wittgenstein's later philosophy changed my understanding of how language works; it shook my view of language's overwhelming and apparent descriptive role. Wittgenstein argued that when discussing any private events – for example, a bodily sensation – we are unable to speak meaningfully as we might speak about a red car, visible to both of us. Ludwig Wittgenstein, *Philosophical Investigations*, Oxford: Basil Blackwell, 2nd edition, 1958 (first published posthumously in English in 1953)

3 Giovanni Maciocia, *The Foundations of Chinese Medicine*, London: Churchill Livingstone, 3rd edition, 2005, pp1171–89

4 This section on habit formation is drawn from James Clear's book, and my experience. James Clear, *Atomic Habits: An Easy and Proven Way to Build Good Habits and Break Bad Ones*, New York: Penguin Random House, 2018

5 Malcom Gladwell, *Talking to Strangers: What we Should Know About People we Don't Know*, London: Allen Lane, 2019

6 VS Ramachandran has multiple videos on the internet which are worth watching. Search specifically for 'Ramachandran, mirror neurons'.

7 VS Ramachandran, *The Tell-Tale Brain: Unlocking the Mystery of Human Nature*, London: Windmill Books, 2012, pp117–135

8 It is interesting that adjacent or close pendulums, even separated by a wall, are known to synchronise over time. So, matching is not just a psychological phenomenon, but also an energetic one. See livescience.com/51644-why-pendulum-clocks-sync-up.html

9 Six months after graduating from the College of Traditional Acupuncture (CTA), near Leamington Spa, I was asked if I could teach a session there. I ended up teaching several weekends in a row and then I supervised a 6-month weekly clinical with 20+ students in a morning. I only later found that my teacher had not been well.

At the time, I responded as if the rapid increase of responsibility was normal. It accelerated my learning and made it obvious that practise and contact with patients was important. I had more practise over that six months than graduates get in a few years. The more patients you see, the more you improve. Multiple comparisons are important. Chinese offspring frequently work for years with their parents – what we would now call 'on the job' training.

10 When I was first in practice, I took my children to an outdoor theme park where we queued for rides. The queue snaked and I was facing a line-up of people about seven or ten feet away. It was a perfect summer's day. I was stunned by seeing facial colours almost leaping off the skin. Afterwards, I never felt satisfied with the poor lighting in most treatment rooms.

11 When I first met my wife Angie, it was early days in terms of learning and we used to get on the London Underground Circle Line and do one circuit just to watch fellow travellers in the opposite seats, then compare notes. Not a good place for colour, but excellent for chronic emotions. On a postgrad course in the US, JR Worsley would take our group to the shopping mall, spot a subject, give us time to observe and later give us feedback.

12 Visit Danny Blyth's website dannyblyth.co.uk and you will find a helpful YouTube video on odour in the 'Acupuncture study' section.

13 There is a lot of agreement that, whether it is 400 or 500 words per minute, we hear much faster than others speak. See livescience.com/60637-listening-enhances-understanding-people-emotions.html

14 Angela and John Hicks, *Healing Your Emotions*, London: Thorsons, 1999, pp12–14

15 A commentator in a 2020 article in a Sunday Times colour supplement said: 'The real problem of humanity is the following: we have Palaeolithic emotions, medieval institutions and godlike technology. And it is terrifically dangerous, and it is now approaching a point of crisis overall.' Edward O Wilson

16 Ekman's discussion can be found in: Daniel Goleman, *Destructive Emotions and How we Can Overcome Them*, London: Bloomsbury, 2004, pp128–137

17 This is sometimes clearly demonstrated on CF days – where practitioners who know their CFs gather in groups and describe what is important to them and what their internal experience is like. The purpose of the day is to understand and respect differences. On occasions, someone will challenge a person who has just spoken to say that they haven't made sense. And it doesn't, at least to the challenger, who is of a different CF.

18 Richard Bandler, *Get the Life you Want: The Secrets to Quick and Lasting Life Change with Neuro-Linguistic Programming*, Florida USA: Health Communications, 2008, pp7–11, and Richard Bandler and Garner Thomson, *The Secrets of Being Happy: The Technology of Hope, Health, and Harmony*, IM Press, 2011, p101–103

19 Paul Eckman and Wallace V Friesen, 'Leaks', *Unmasking the Face*, Major Books, Cambridge MA, 2009, pp144–45

20 I learned this from an NLP trainer called Michael Grinder, who showed me the value of slowing things down for understanding group interactions, and then in a private session the benefits of using slowed video for not missing what I have called 'leaks'.

21 For example, David Pickering, *Pocket Jokes*, London: Penguin Books, 2006, or Geoff Tibballs, *The Mammoth Book of One-Liners*, London: Constable and Robinson, 2012. For someone who used not so easily to slip into joy, I groan over nine one-liners and then the tenth makes me smile, snigger, chuckle or burst out laughing. 'What's the cure for water on the knee. A tap on the ankle.'

22 In the *Bible*, when someone was to 'gird up their loins,' they were to do so in preparation to run, fight, or do hard labour. So, basically, it means 'get ready' or 'man up'. 'Gird up now thy loins like a man; for I will demand of thee, and answer thou me.' The *Bible* (aside from being sexist) expressed the idea of rising to a difficult situation.

23 A group exercise is to create a line-up of five people in front of the rest of the group, one of each CF, and then for group members to arrange them left to right with the person with the least movement in the Upper Burner on the left and the next least beside that person, and so on. Metal CFs invariably end up on the left. It is a subtle observation but it clearly has a basis. You may be able to find somewhere in public where you can observe the breathing of someone, who is not talking.

24 Angela and John Hicks, *Healing Your Emotions*, London: Thorsons, 1999, pp147–153. This account is based on that incident and is a clear and strong suggestion for Metal CFs.

25 In *Healing Your Emotions*, it is recommended that Metal CFs formulate and give positive inner qualities (PIQs) to others to assist their being able to take in PIQs. My own experience, as a patient and Metal CF was that expressing PIQs to others was not easy, but made a big difference, and I believe made the treatment I received more effective.

26 Giovanni Maciocia, *The Foundations of Chinese Medicine*, London: Churchill Livingstone, 3rd edition, 2005, p599

27 I rarely noticed this leakage of fear until I made videos of some Water CFs and played them back one frame at a time, 25 frames per second. I then saw clearly that with some 'lack of fear' Water CFs, fear leaked out, but so rapidly I missed it. When you carry out such a test, you need to be fluent and hyper-alert (see Chapter 13, page 106 on slow-motion emotion testing). It is, however, enough to observe in response to you being scary, the apparent lack of fear.

28 In the 20th century, existentialist philosophy has arisen and states that man exists first and has no essential nature, whereas previously Western philosophers were endlessly trying to define man's essence. I may be wrong, but I think Chinese philosophers did try to define man's essence, but remained more practical.

29 This is a paraphrase of an advertisement for a breakfast cereal: 'Wheaties – the Breakfast of Champions'.

30 John Cassidy and BC Rimbeaux, *Juggling for the Complete Klutz*, Palo Alto, California: Klutz Press, 4th edition, 1994 is an enjoyable account of how to juggle following the same principles.

31 Jackie Shaw, Penelope Bidgood and Nasrollah Saebi, 'Exploring acupuncture outcomes in a college clinic', *European Journal of Oriental Medicine (EJOM)*, 2007, Vol 5(4), pp55–63

Acknowledgements

To my original teacher, JR Worsley, who initiated the acupuncture phase of my life for which I am grateful and which made the dream of helping others through acupuncture treatment a most satisfying commitment.

To Angie, my wife, for love, companionship and support, and for sharing the initial creation of the College of Integrated Chinese Medicine (CICM), Reading, UK.

To those who were readers, advisors and supporters as this book came together, including Sharon Ashton, Danny Blyth, Kim Chan, Angie Hicks, Greg Lampert, Bill Mueller, Jonathan Pledger and Ehsan Salout.

To all my neuro-linguistic programming (NLP) teachers and colleagues who made modelling a fascinating part of my life.

To my fellow teachers at CICM who have shared the challenges and pleasure of teaching Five Element constitutional acupuncture integrated with Traditional Chinese Medicine (TCM).

To the students of both Acupuncture Training Courses and CICM who developed sensory acuity and integration skills and inspired me to write this book.

To those who attended Thursday evening sensory acuity classes at CICM.

To Bridget Long, a massive thank you for editing and formatting the book, working in collaboration with her family, Beatty, Sam and David. Her support and commitment to putting it together has made it coherent, and beautiful.

Expressions of emotion on the face and body tend to be a continuum, and are often fleeting. These change processes are hard to capture in a single still image, so follow the descriptions rather than the illustrations, and learn to identify emotions in real life.

Senses and sensitivity: The 'doing' of Five Element constitutional acupuncture
First edition © John Hicks, 2023

ISBN 978-1-3999-5411-2

Design and book production Bridget Long, Sam Hallas and David Hallas
Illustrations © Beatty Hallas, 2023
Faces pp39, 99, 123 © Shutterstock